3/00

✓

The
Antidepressant
Survival
Program

The Antidepressant Survival Program

How to Beat the Side Effects and Enhance the Benefits of Your Medication

ROBERT J. HEDAYA, M.D.
with Deborah Kotz

A Living Planet Book

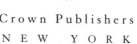

Crown Publishers
NEW YORK

This book is not intended to substitute for consultation with a qualified medical doctor. The author recommends consultation with a medical doctor before beginning any part of the program. The author or his agents will not accept responsibility for injury, loss, or damage occasioned to any person acting or refraining from action as a result of material in this book, whether or not such injury, loss, or damage is due in any way to any negligent act or omission, breach of duty, or default on the part of the author or his agents.

For the sake of privacy, the names of the patients whose stories are told in this book and personal details that might identify them have been changed.

Published by Crown Publishers, 201 East 50th Street, New York, New York 10022. Member of the Crown Publishing Group.

Random House, Inc. New York, Toronto, London, Sydney, Auckland
www.randomhouse.com

Crown is a trademark and the Crown colophon is a registered trademark of Random House, Inc.

DESIGN BY LYNNE AMFT

Printed in the United States of America

Library of Congress Cataloging-in-Publication Data
Hedaya, Robert J.
The antidepressant survival program : how to beat the side effects and enhance the benefits of your medication / Robert J. Hedaya.
Includes bibliographical references.
1. Antidepressants. 2. Antidepressants—Side effects. 3. Psychopharmacology. 4. Depression, Mental. I. Title.
RM332 .H43 2000
616.85'27061—dc21   99-33924
                                                             CIP

ISBN 0-609-60465-1

10 9 8 7 6 5 4 3 2 1

First Edition

To Life!

Contents

THE MEDICAL PRESCRIPTION

Foreword

Despite the tremendous advances in the treatment of depression in recent years, many patients, even with the best medical care, feel that they are not living rich and fulfilling lives. These are the so-called partial responders. For others the side effects of their medications have paradoxically created new obstacles to reclaiming the daily pleasures that they have lost to depression.

Bob Hedaya is one of those rare doctors who has been able to bring a broad range of skills to bear on solving the problem of side effects (including unwanted weight gain, lethargy, and loss of sexual vitality) as well as incomplete responses to antidepressant medication.

Bob's open-mindedness, on the one hand, and respect for hard-nosed science, on the other, are unusual among medical doctors. In this age of superspecialization, physicians can easily be hemmed in by their narrow fields of research, which is why an out-of-the-box thinker like Bob is so valuable. He brings a comprehensive knowledge of divergent fields to bear on any problem, from nutrition and fitness to psychopharmacology and endocrinology. In this book, he offers a wealth of wisdom drawn from years of clinical experience, research, and teaching.

The Antidepressant Survival Program is a much-needed lantern in the darkness: a beacon of hope, a prescription for health. The program Bob presents in this book is a marriage of creativity and pragmatism. It draws on important new research from a wide range of disciplines that impact the mind and the body, while managing to avoid being doctrinaire. As he says in his introduction, whatever's safe and effective is in play. Rather than taking the easy route of damning antidepressant medications as worse than the cure—and they emphatically are not—he's devised a comprehensive program for *maximizing the benefits of antidepressants while minimizing their side effects.*

But what I suspect most readers will appreciate in Bob's book is his wisdom. His approach is as simple as it is compassionate: patients can have the best of both worlds—freedom from depression *and* freedom from side effects. Unlike doctors who might adopt the attitude "Be thankful you're not depressed anymore," Bob has a far broader goal in mind: a full life, with self-esteem, body image, vitality, and sexuality intact.

The program outlined in this book—based on his years of clinical experience—is very ambitious. It offers people not just a remedy for side effects, but a chance to make a *full recovery* from symptoms to enjoy a level of physical and psychological health they may never have experienced before.

In his excellent previous book, *Understanding Biological Psychiatry,* Bob speaks to colleagues with interest in the biological aspects of mental health. In *The Antidepressant Survival Program* he speaks directly to the patient who suffers not only from the pain of incomplete medication response, but also from the pain-in-the-neck side effects that go with antidepressant treatments.

I have known Bob in many capacities—as a trusted friend, a valued colleague, a fellow researcher at the National Institute of Mental Health, and a faculty member of Georgetown University. For years, his patients have been the beneficiaries of his progressive and comprehensive approach to healing. Now everyone, patients and doctors alike, can reap the rewards of his work.

Norman E. Rosenthal, M.D.
Clinical Professor of Psychiatry
Georgetown University
Washington, D.C.

The
Antidepressant
Survival
Program

"I'm Not Depressed Anymore, but When Do I Get a Life?"

* * *

LIKE MOST PSYCHIATRISTS, I was tremendously excited by the advent of Prozac and other selective serotonin reuptake inhibitor (SSRI) antidepressants in the late 1980s. These drugs were hailed as medical miracles, and in many ways they were. Compared with conventional psychotherapy and existing medications, this new category of drugs seemed to promise salvation from the ravages of depression—as well as a host of nondepressive disorders—with negligible side effects.

But like many "wonder drugs," SSRI antidepressants have proven to be a mixed blessing. For the majority of depressed people, these medications offer a desperately needed bridge back from crippling and sometimes suicidal despair. *But these same lifesaving drugs confront patients with daunting roadblocks to full recovery in the form of serious side effects—such as physical and mental lethargy, loss of sex drive and performance, and significant weight gain.*

These side effects erode the fragile wellness and self-esteem that you, or someone you care about, have been working so hard to rebuild. Faced with such fundamental impediments to their health and happiness, many people taking antidepressants become discouraged and stop taking their medication—usually with the calamitous result of renewed symptoms.

Sadly, many doctors do not appreciate, or may even dismiss, their patients' complaints about side effects. "You're so much better than you were before you started on medication," they insist, encouraging patients to accept the lesser of two evils. "Every drug has side effects. You'll just have to learn to live with them," they counsel.

Not only does this all-too-common response lack compassion but it's bad medicine. By dismissing antidepressants' side effects as something they must learn to live with, doctors are forfeiting their patients' chance to fully reclaim their lives—and their happiness—from the shadow of depression.

If a primary symptom of depression is an inability to enjoy life, then finding pleasure in relationships and work is the ultimate goal of recovery. Who among us can expect to be desirable to others if we feel undesirable? How can we expect to fully enjoy the pleasures of intimacy without a healthy sex drive, full sexual function, or a positive body image? Who can hope to compete on the fast track of life and work with reduced vitality and mental alertness?

These questions are hardly peripheral concerns; they go to the heart of recovery from depression. The truth is, we can't embrace life at arm's length, and we can't love life without loving ourselves.

GETTING A LIFE

For years I treated patients for depression, with both psychotherapy and drugs, only to find their progress impeded by new sets of obstacles. They gained weight—sometimes so much that they resigned themselves to the sidelines of social life. (More frequently, they stopped taking their medication and soon relapsed into depression.)[1] Their sex

---

[1] Since antidepressant medications are used to treat a wide range of conditions (listed on page 4), I will refer to depression as the main symptom, though any number of conditions may apply.

drives deserted them—love relationships and marriages foundered amid sexual apathy and dysfunction. Most critically, they lacked the energy to keep up with their jobs and fully engage the everyday challenges of life.

Over and over again, I heard the same refrain from these patients: "I'm not depressed anymore, but I'm still not fully enjoying the things that are most important to me: my work, my love life, myself. When do I get a life?"

Whether because of stubbornness, pride, or perhaps some loftier motive, I could never walk away from a patient until his or her problems were solved. As I got more deeply involved in difficult, "treatment-resistant" cases of depression and chronic fatigue syndrome, I realized I would have to expand my search for solutions. I knew that a lot of recent research in the basic sciences hadn't made its way from the researchers' lab benches to the clinicians and patients who needed it most. Drawing on my background in psychiatry, general medicine, and psychopharmacology, I examined the latest literature for any new research that might shed light on these problems. Then, through trial and error, I gradually uncovered their remedies.

The result of this multidisciplinary investigation is the Antidepressant Survival Program. Now when a new patient asks me, "Does the treatment for depression have to be worse than the disease?" my answer is a resolute "No!"

The positive results achieved by well over three hundred patients in my practice confirm this promise. Their success rate for reducing, and in most cases eliminating, the harmful side effects of antidepressant medication has astounded me—80 to 90 percent of patients who faithfully follow the program achieve the desired result. Even more gratifying, my patients have found that my Antidepressant Survival Program actually enhances the therapeutic benefits of their medications, while reducing or eliminating their side effects.

Over time more and more people have come to me for help. Meanwhile, more and more doctors have begun referring patients to me. It became clear that many patients on antidepressants simply weren't getting meaningful help for their side effects from their physicians.

That's why I decided to translate my program into a book. In the following chapters you will learn how to free yourself from your medication's side effects while remaining free from depression. I believe—and my clinical practice has proven—that *no one* should have to be resigned to half a life, simply because he or she is on antidepressant medication. *Everyone* recovering from depression should aspire to the happiness and fulfillment that comes with vitality, a positive body image, a healthy sex life—and the higher-quality relationships these things foster.

THE PROMISE AND PROBLEM OF ANTIDEPRESSANTS

Over 25 million Americans are currently on antidepressant medication, *because it's the best option available to them.* For mild to severe depression, SSRI antidepressants (Prozac, Paxil, Luvox, Celexa, and Zoloft are the most commonly used, though there are many others) and Wellbutrin and Serzone offer relief with the fewest side effects, compared with previously available drugs. And millions of other patients have discovered that SSRIs provide relief from a wide range of *nondepressive* disorders, including

Generalized anxiety disorder
Panic disorder
Obsessive-compulsive spectrum disorders
Fibromyalgia
Premenstrual syndrome (PMS)
Chronic pain syndrome
Irritable bowel syndrome
Migraine headaches
Chronic fatigue–immune dysfunction syndrome
Substance abuse and addiction
Posttraumatic stress syndrome
Anorexia nervosa
Bulimia nervosa

What about so-called natural remedies? A lot has been written recently about the "miracle" of St. John's wort. Indeed, this herb helps people cope with mild to moderate depression. But it doesn't work for many depressed people, particularly if their condition is moderate to severe. Further, St. John's wort has troublesome side effects of its own, and unlike SSRIs, St. John's wort has no proven therapeutic effect on the nondepressive disorders just mentioned. (Also, quality control of many St. John's wort preparations is uneven.)

Unfortunately, antidepressants aren't a panacea.

As the initial euphoria over SSRI antidepressants subsided, both patients and their doctors began to realize just how widespread their side effects were. It is now clear that up to 80 percent of patients on SSRI antidepressant medications experience side effects such as lethargy, weight gain, and loss of libido (and many of these go unreported because of the stigma associated with sexual dysfunction). Depending on the survey and the side effects being reported, anywhere from 30 to 80 percent of patients on SSRI medication suffer side effects so severe that they are significantly impaired in their ability to function in their jobs or relationships.

The medical underpinnings of side effects are complex and not fully understood, but this much is clear: *Antidepressants are powerful agents that cause widespread changes in the body's neurochemical and hormonal systems.* When one of the body's metabolic systems is altered, this tends to create disequilibrium in others—which is, in part, why so many people suffer from multiple side effects.

When it comes to coping with these disturbing side effects, most people are on their own. It's not that their doctors aren't caring people. They simply lack the expertise to respond constructively to their patients' complaints. The majority of psychiatrists have only a rudimentary knowledge of psychopharmacology—and even less understanding of the related fields of endocrinology, nutrition, immunology, and gastroenterology. And with the growth of managed care, more and more people are being prescribed antidepressants by their primary-care physicians, who have no psychiatric expertise and very little understanding of how these drugs are affecting their patients. Even those doctors who take their patients' complaints to heart have little to offer beyond a change in medication, which is often only a partial solution to the problem.

THE SOLUTION: RESTORING BALANCE
TO YOUR BODY AND LIFE

Thanks to recent medical progress, the biochemistry governing antidepressant side effects—particularly weight gain, loss of sexuality, and decreased mental acuity—is gradually coming to be understood. These side effects are the results of specific, usually treatable imbalances in the brain and body. You will see that this program employs a wide range of treatment modes—nutrition and exercise, hormonal and herbal supplements, meditation and much more—to redress the imbalances caused by medication and reestablish healthful function.

There is no simple, one-size-fits-all remedy for side effects, because every person responds differently to antidepressant medications. Every person's body is different. But nearly everyone can benefit from my program because its goal is the same for all people: to diagnose and counteract the imbalances in the body.

When imbalance occurs, the body struggles to compensate and to reassert its natural balance and healthy order. This innate drive toward equilibrium is your body's hidden gift. Antidepressants are powerful agents. Overcoming their negative side effects is not and cannot be effortless. But as you draw nearer and nearer the rewarding life you seek, this wellness program, in collaboration with your body's innate drive to heal itself, will prove to be a surprisingly unstoppable force for recovery.

Mine is an integrative, holistic approach that incorporates recent breakthroughs in psychopharmacology, nutrition, immunology, gastroenterology, and endocrinology—what I call Whole Psychiatry. Rather than getting bogged down in meaningless distinctions between "natural" and "traditional" treatments, this program is guided by two simple and pragmatic questions: Is it safe? and Does it work?

It *is* safe. The danger to most patients lies in going off their medication; 80 percent of people who have had more than two depressive episodes will relapse within one year if they stop taking their medication.

And it works. More than three hundred patients have proven that *all* motivated individuals can enjoy increased self-esteem, confidence, vitality, vigor, and sex drive—in short, a level of healthfulness they may never have experienced before.

My program is grounded in the basic principle of returning the body's natural healthfulness and balance. Specifically, it

* Restores the vital biological factors—including micronutrients (e.g., vitamins, minerals, amino acids, and essential fatty acids) and hormones—that are often depleted and are essential to the body's health
* Restores the optimal function and proper balance of the body's metabolic and energy systems
* Restores the ability to experience pleasure in life (inability to experience pleasure is a classic symptom of depression)
* Restores the crucial balance among work, stress, and play

This program is for anyone who believes, as I do, that it's not enough to survive depression. *You can thrive.* Since you're reading this book, I probably don't have to convince you that there's a fuller, more satisfying life than the one you have.

So, do yourself a favor. Get a life!

CHAPTER ONE

The Antidepressant Survival Program in a Nutshell

An Integrative Approach to Eliminating the Side Effects and Enhancing the Benefits of Antidepressants

* * *

On every crossway on the road that leads to the future, each progressive spirit is opposed by a thousand men appointed to guard the past.

MAURICE MAETERLINCK

MY ANTIDEPRESSANT SURVIVAL PROGRAM began to take shape in 1983, when I became frustrated by the failure of antidepressants and cognitive therapy to alleviate fully the depression of Donna, a thirty-five-year-old single woman who had been my patient for over a year. Donna had tried a combination of tricyclic and monoamine oxidase (MAO) inhibitor antidepressants—this was before Prozac, Wellbutrin, Serzone, and additional selective serotonin reuptake inhibitors (SSRIs) came onto the market. Yet she was still feeling depressed and lethargic

9

to the extent that she couldn't function in her daily life. Not only weren't the medications helping her depression, they were making her feel extremely tired throughout the day.

The evening before Donna came in for one of her sessions, I read and reread her chart to see if I could figure out what I was missing. In the notes about her medical history, I noticed that Donna had irregular menstrual periods. That symptom, combined with her fatigue and the fact that she was overweight and very sensitive to cold temperatures, suggested to me that she could have an underactive thyroid system, a condition that can cause depressed moods, lethargy, and weight gain—and that can actually be *caused by* antidepressant medications. I had already done the routine screening test for this condition, and the result was normal, but the symptoms were at odds with the laboratory results.

I read up on the thyroid system. I began to understand that this routine screening test was not a complete evaluation of the thyroid system (although it was the medical standard of the time). I decided to have Donna's thyroid evaluated more thoroughly. My suspicion was correct—Donna had an underactive thyroid, which I remedied with supplemental thyroid hormone. Two weeks after Donna's thyroid condition was treated, her lethargy and weight gain began to lessen, and soon she felt happier and more energetic than she had in years.

After my experience with Donna, I became preoccupied by two questions that have shaped my psychiatric practice ever since: First, how many other patients had physiological imbalances that resulted from their use of antidepressants? Second, how many of my patients were suffering from undiagnosed, hidden conditions that masqueraded as psychiatric conditions or medication side effects, or at the least contributed to their symptoms? I began to take much more extensive medical histories and perform physical exams. I also began to use more medical tests to check for hidden health conditions that could have been caused by the antidepressants or could be hindering the medications' therapeutic effects. I began to appreciate more fully the link between the mind and body and came to this realization: *I could not heal the mind without simultaneously healing the body.*

Remember, this was back in the mid-1980s. The notion of a mind-body connection was still viewed with much skepticism by the mainstream medical world, and many doctors believed alternative medicine was quackery. I was putting myself out on a limb, and I have to admit even I had many doubts about this uncharted territory. Was I making too great a leap by searching for undiagnosed illnesses in patients who did not respond to antidepressants or had troubling side effects? I questioned myself every step of the way, but I knew that my medical detective work was better than the alternative, simply telling my patients, "There's nothing more I can do. You'll just have to learn to live with the side effects of antidepressants," or "This is the best relief you can expect from your condition."

My doubts were repeatedly put to rest when patients who seemed stuck in a limbo of dysfunction suddenly recovered vital and fully functional lives. Meanwhile, my increasing understanding of physiology and science from a broad range of fields convinced me that treating these problems demanded a much broader diagnostic and therapeutic lens.

As a doctor, I was never very comfortable prescribing a drug unless I was prepared to help my patients deal with its side effects. Gradually, being the integrative thinker that I am, I came to see myself as a conductor who tuned and harmonized the various instruments within the vast orchestra of my patients' minds and bodies. By prescribing antidepressants, I knew I could tune those orchestra sections of the mind that are responsible for stabilizing moods and lifting depression, panic, or anxiety. At the same time, however, antidepressants all too frequently introduced new disharmonies, throwing other parts of the orchestra out of tune—causing problems such as hormone imbalances and sexual dysfunction. In order to restore optimal balance and harmony between these systems, I had to make some sense out of the cacophony, then figure out how to retune each section of the orchestra.

I came to the conclusion that there is no single answer. Unfortunately, there was no one pill I could prescribe to wipe out the side effects of antidepressants. (Even if there were, I'd probably need yet another pill to wipe out the side effects from the second one, and so on.) My fascination with these interlocking biosystems led me to study the basic research relevant to both the side effects of antidepressants and the medical problems my patients were experiencing. Gradually, I found ways to offset the imbalances created by antidepressants—as well as correct the underlying disorders that the medications made worse.

As time went on I began to realize that these two intertwined issues—alleviating the side effects of antidepressants and uncovering and treating hidden medical disorders—required more than medical tests and drug treatments. During the early 1990s it became clear to me that nutrition, exercise, and other lifestyle factors all played roles in combating the side effects of antidepressants while bolstering the medications' benefits. (As has often been the case in medicine, clinicians on the front lines were finding out what worked ahead of the researchers. Over the past three or four years, research studies have been confirming what I discovered in my practice.) I formulated nutrition, exercise, and stress management plans that became the foundation of my program—what I call the Fundamentals. The Fundamentals are based on sound, tested medical principles that will improve your overall health and alleviate antidepressant side effects while amplifying the therapeutic value of the antidepressants. I then combined the Fundamentals with my diagnostic tests, which I call the Medical Prescription, to create the Antidepressant Survival Program.

The Antidepressant Survival Program has one overriding goal: *To create healthy, balanced functioning in both your body and your mind, which will enable you to live your life as you were meant to live it: with energy, excitement, pleasure, and vitality. A balanced body and mind are the keys to recapturing the joys and freedoms that make life worth living—the ability to create and experience the simple but profound pleasures of love, work, and play.*

This may seem like a pretty lofty goal, but it is, I assure you, one that is well worth pursuing. As with anything of value in life, it requires a clear commitment. And as with anything else in life, you will get out of it what you put into it. What, exactly, do you need to commit to? You must become an active partner in your medical care. You must understand that you are the *creator* of your health. This means rethinking your eating habits and shedding your perhaps sedentary ways. You will also need to actively find pleasures to counterbalance your daily stresses. And you will have to forge a strong partnership with your doctor to diagnose and treat any hidden health problems that may have been caused by your depression, or resulted from taking antidepressants. (And if you're in therapy, you may want to ask your therapist to help coach you through the program.)

Your first thought might be, I'm just not at a point in my life where I can make major changes. That is understandable. After all, change requires energy, a resource that you may feel you can't spare if you're taking antidepressants. Making matters worse, your day is probably already overloaded; you may be working hard to get a promotion or agonizing over how to arrange car pools around your kids' frenetic schedules. Between the laundry that's piling up, the bathroom that hasn't been cleaned in weeks, the dentist appointment that you haven't had time to make, you're probably asking yourself: How can I possibly fit even one more thing into my jam-packed life?

Many of my patients have asked me the same question. I tell them, "Just take the first step. After only a few days you'll begin to *feel* the rewards of this program. Your motivation will follow naturally." I've devised a motivational Five-Day Jump Start (see Chapter 3) that will help you overcome inertia and build momentum.

The good news is that this program is self-reinforcing: the rewards of each stage motivate you toward the next. The negative forces that normally hold you in a state of slow motion will turn into a momentum that propels you forward.

The Antidepressant Survival Program will give you your life back. It won't eliminate your work or household duties, but it will make these responsibilities less daunting, since your increased energy will make you much more efficient. Patients have told me that they're amazed at how much they can accomplish in one day without energy slumps to drag them down. This is just one of the tangible rewards.

The Antidepressant Survival Program will help you lose the excess pounds that you may have put on as a result of going through depression or taking antidepressants—and maintain a healthy weight. And once you have integrated the program into your lifestyle, the weight will stay off. This is a second tangible reward.

The program is also designed to renew your sexual energies, which may have been drained from your previous symptoms or from your use of antidepressants. You'll find that you have more desire to have sex, that you'll have an easier time achieving orgasm, and that sex will be more pleasurable overall. This is a third tangible reward.

But there are also rewards that are less tangible. As I was writing this chapter, I received a call from a patient who had been following my program for about two months. "Dr. Hedaya, I can't believe the energy I feel," she told me. Others have said that they feel better than they've ever felt in their lives. One sixty-six-year-old woman tells me she has more energy now than she had when she was in her twenties.

Renewable, self-sustaining energy, increased pleasure and fun, a renewed sense of freedom, a healthy body weight, a blossoming of sexuality. These gifts to yourself will transform the tenor of your life and renew your spirit. How would you like to wake up in the morning with energy and enthusiasm for the day? How would you like to look in the mirror and feel good about yourself? How would you like to feel in control of your body and your life, instead of indentured to side effects that take a heavy daily toll?

Let me give you a brief overview of my program, which I'll explain in more detail in the coming chapters. Here are the main ingredients:

The Fundamentals: nutrition, exercise, and spiritual renewal
(including play and stress reduction)

The Medical Prescription: hormones, gut reactions, and
sexual renewal

THE FUNDAMENTALS
A BALANCED NUTRITION PLAN

Good nutrition is fundamentally important to all people but particularly to people on antidepressants for several reasons. Adequate protein is essential for producing the brain's all-important neurotransmitters, which help stabilize moods. Amino acids, essential fats, vitamins, and minerals are also necessary to allow antidepressants to do their job. And good nutrition helps control blood-sugar levels, which reduces irritability, anxiety, moodiness, fatigue, and excess weight, not to mention a host of other symptoms. Furthermore, as body fat decreases, blood flow is improved to the brain and the genitals, enhancing both mental processes and sexual responsiveness.

The nutrition plan lists foods that are toxic for people who take antidepressants because they fuel unhealthy food cravings, deplete physical and sexual energy, and encourage weight gain. Foods such as sugar, refined flour, caffeine, chocolate, and alcohol are slow-acting poisons. All contribute to the side effects of antidepressants.

On the flip side, my nutrition plan increases your intake of medicinal foods that will help alleviate side effects and actually make the antidepressants work better. This list includes protein-rich foods, those with "good" fats (omega-3 essential fatty acids and monounsaturated fats), and the healing, *unprocessed* foods present in nature (whole grains, fruits, seeds, and vegetables).

The primary goal of the nutrition plan is eating healthy foods in the right balance. Weight loss is not the main goal of the plan, but, particularly in combination with my exercise program and the Medical Prescription program, it will help you lose weight and regain your youthful proportions. *My nutrition plan is not a deprivation diet.* I *don't* want you to become a nutrition fanatic. I *don't* want you to restrict your calories or count fat grams. I'm *not* asking you to cut down on your portion sizes. Eat as much as you like. What I'm offering is a healthful eating program that will help you shed pounds by banishing your cravings for sweets and starchy foods.

I'll ask you to keep track of the foods you eat in a food diary and to think in advance about how you're going to implement certain changes in your eating habits. Most of my patients change their eating habits gradually, over several weeks or even months. Coming to terms with the effects of harmful foods is an incremental process. Most people can't reinvent their nutritional habits completely on day one. You will find, however, that as you eat fewer and fewer toxic foods, you will crave them less and less.

As you shift the balance away from poisonous foods toward medicinal ones, you will naturally begin to desire an appropriate balance of protein to carbohydrates. My basic rule of thumb is to fill your plate with roughly one-third protein-rich foods (meat, chicken, fish, tofu) and two-thirds carbohydrates (fruits and complex carbohydrates such as beans, whole grains, and most vegetables). This is based on research that has found that adequate amounts of certain amino acids (the building blocks of protein) are essential for manufacturing brain chemicals such as serotonin and dopamine—which help regulate numerous mind-body functions, such as mood, pleasure, energy, appetite, sexual performance, and hormonal and gastrointestinal function. Adequate amounts of protein (as well as other nutrients) are essential for antidepressants to do their job. This balance of protein to carbohydrates (with a sufficient amount of the good kind of fat) is also essential for stabilizing blood-sugar levels—which are a major cause of food cravings, depleted energy levels, irritability, poor concentration, daytime sleepiness, and even anxiety and blue moods.

The more diligent you are about incorporating the nutrition plan into your life, the more energetic you'll feel and the more successful you'll be at taking off any unwanted weight you gained on antidepressants (while you reshape your body through exercise and the Medical Prescription plan).

Foods found in nature are not as exciting to our jaded palates as the processed poisons we have grown accustomed to. Our natural taste for good food has been co-opted by sugar, salt, artificial flavorings, and myriad "other ingredients" added to virtually all the processed foods we eat. To make the transition from processed poisons and excess pounds to normal food and weight, this nutrition plan helps retrain your taste buds toward healthful foods. (Meanwhile, other elements of the program will help you develop complementary sources of pleasure, including athletic activity, play, and sex.) As you wean yourself off the toxic foods that worsen your antidepressant side effects, they will gradually lose their appeal. Once you begin fueling your body with the proper nutrition, *all* of your body's systems and functions will improve. You'll feel more energetic and alert, *and* you'll feel the beneficial effects of the antidepressants with greater intensity.

A Balanced Exercise Program

Exercise plays a major role in combating antidepressant side effects. It increases circulation, bringing more oxygen to the brain and other organs. And exercise serves other purposes as well. When you're exercising properly, your appetite begins to reflect the appropriate needs of your body. Excesses of appetite—the very excesses that most antidepressants cause—are curbed. And, like good nutrition, vigorous exercise heightens the effectiveness of your antidepressant medication.

The exercise program works in concert with the nutrition plan to help you reshape your body, lose fat, renew your energy, and build strength. I do not believe it is possible to regain your normal body proportions by dietary changes alone. So my program includes the three essential elements of good fitness: a healthy heart via aerobic exercise, strong muscles via strength training, and flexibility via stretching exercises. Keeping in mind that everyone is at a different fitness level, I've developed a three-stage program that allows you to enter at your current level of fitness and gradually work up from there.

During Stage 1, which lasts for six weeks, you'll learn to master one type of steady or aerobic exercise and you'll become comfortable with strength training and stretching. During Stage 2, which also lasts for six weeks, you'll focus on cross training by incorporating two new aerobic activities into your workouts. This will enable you to work different muscle groups and to build some variety into your workouts, preparing you for Stage 3. Stage 3 focuses on maintaining your exercise program and, more important, helping your exercise become a source of fun, pleasure, and even spiritual renewal.

The exercise program specifically works with the nutrition plan to minimize antidepressant side effects. Of course, exercise burns fat and builds muscle, thereby working hand in hand with the nutrition plan to help you lose weight. Moreover, it curbs your appetite and helps regulate blood-sugar levels to tame your cravings. By improving your circulation, exercise helps deliver the nutrients from the foods you eat to your brain and other organs. Exercise also triggers the release of feel-good hormones, which improve your mood. In addition, you will notice that your sex life improves thanks to increased circulation, which heightens arousal and sensitivity in your sex organs. Perhaps most important, exercise will improve your body image and make you feel better about yourself as you take steps to a healthier life.

STRESS REDUCTION, PLAY, AND SPIRITUAL RENEWAL

It is, perhaps, a sad testament to our spiritually impoverished culture that we actually need to have a plan to revive the spirit. But I've found that relaxation, play, and spirituality are frequently missing from my patients' lives. Minimizing stress and maximizing fun are crucial to experiencing pleasure. All the medical treatments, food, and exercise in the world won't do you much good if you're too stressed out to enjoy yourself.

From a scientific standpoint, learning to relax, play, and tap into your spirituality will help normalize your body's production of stress hormones while boosting its production of pleasure chemicals, like endorphins and dopamine. *This effect has an undeniably major role in weight management.* It can help you feel happy, energized, and sexually recharged. Relaxation techniques have been found to have a powerful normalizing effect on the stress-hormone-producing adrenal glands, which frequently go out of balance in people who have suffered from depression. Renewing your spiritual life has a similar effect and, according to much research, may actually help you live longer and healthier. Remember that play and fun were once essential parts of your life. Experiencing the joy of spontaneity, novelty, creativity, and curiosity exercises the pleasure-producing dopamine and endorphin pathways.

Relaxation, play, and spiritual renewal might strike you as "soft" concerns compared with hormonal and dietary imbalances. In fact, they go to the heart of my program, because they promote healthy brain and hormone functions, and they are vital to reconnecting with aspects of your life you may have lost to depression or antidepressants. *It's impossible to recover a fulfilling life without access to contentment and joy.*

THE MEDICAL PRESCRIPTION

While the Fundamentals can be done on your own, or with a therapist or a supportive friend as coach, the Medical Prescription part of my program requires you to work closely with your doctor. He or she will diagnose and treat any hidden medical problems that may be throwing your body out of balance—even if you are already following the Fundamental components of the program. The Medical Prescription is tailored to your own medical needs. The beginning of every section includes quizzes to clue you in to whether you may have a particular health problem that should be investigated by your doctor. You'll see that these chapters also contain Notes to Your Doctor, which detail some of the medical science and give my recommendations for diagnostic tests and treatments.

Evaluating the Hormone Connection

Hormones are among the most important regulatory agents in the body. When they are not in proper balance, wide-ranging dysfunction results. The brain, gastrointestinal tract, thyroid, pancreas, and adrenal and parathyroid glands all secrete powerful hormones, each with far-reaching consequences for health and normal functioning.

Hormonal balance is critical to treating depression. The brain cannot function in a normal way if hormones are not present and released in proper amounts at the proper times. Other negative consequences will be felt throughout the body. For instance, it's a little-known fact that antidepressants can reduce normal thyroid function. This sets off a chain reaction of health consequences, causing the body to function in a type of slow motion; most people experience weight gain, lethargy, and mental fatigue, in addition to many other symptoms. These symptoms are often misdiagnosed as mere "side effects" of the antidepressant and receive no specific treatment.

Even more common are adrenal system malfunctions, which affect about 80 percent of my patients. Adrenal system abnormalities frequently arise during depression, which puts your body into a chronic state of stress. And they may linger even after depression seems to lift and can contribute to antidepressant side effects by making you feel tired and depleted of energy, as well as contributing to weight gain and reduced sex drive.

Dealing with Gut Reactions

A broad spectrum of negative gut reactions can rob your body of the vital nutrients it needs to manufacture neurotransmitters, hormones, and other chemicals necessary to healing depression and eliminating side effects. Without these nutrients, you can still feel depressed even if you're on high doses of medication. So you could be following the nutrition plan to the letter but not feeling your best if your body isn't properly digesting and absorbing the foods you eat. You may find that you still feel excessively tired or drained of energy or that you have a general sense of malaise. Your problems could be the result of a food sensitivity or digestive abnormality, or perhaps you have a condition that causes low blood sugar. These are all part of the gut reactions that are common in people who experience side effects.

The first line of action I recommend is a series of blood tests to measure the levels of certain vitamins, minerals, and other nutrients in your blood. These will indicate to your doctor whether you are deficient in any essential nutrients. Sometimes a supplement is all that is needed, but your doctor should rule out any underlying causes that may be preventing your body from absorbing these nutrients. I recommend what I think are the best tests for diagnosing the problem. All the tests are noninvasive, but some need to be performed by certain labs to obtain the most reliable results. (I explain this in the Note to Your Doctor sections.) Some tests are self-evaluations: If you or your doctor suspects a food sensitivity, for instance, I recommend going on a food elimination diet. In this case, you will temporarily abstain from particular foods and see how you feel. In investigating digestive problems that are common in patients who use antidepressants, the main goal is to determine whether the body is deficient in certain nutrients, why it is deficient, and what treatment will reverse the deficiency.

Reclaiming Your Sexual Vitality

A diminished sex life is one of the most common—yet least discussed—antidepressant side effects. You may experience partial or complete impotence, or an inability to achieve orgasm. Others experience subtler effects, like a diminished desire for sex or less pleasure during sex, and they wonder if their relationships have gone sour or if they're just too stressed out. In this section of the program, you will learn how to solve the vast array of sexual problems that frequently result from taking antidepressants. (But keep in mind that the other parts of the program often help solve sexual problems as well.)

I will walk you through a four-step process to help you reclaim your sexual vitality. As you move through the steps (assessing your sex hormone levels, adjusting your antidepressants, exploring various pharmaceutical, hormonal, or herbal remedies), you can stop on a particular step if you find that it is working for you. Viagra, the highly publicized pill for impotence, gets a special mention. I've found it to be extraordinarily helpful in overcoming erectile dysfunction caused by antidepressants. Viagra may also prove useful in women to heighten both arousal and sexual pleasure. The goal of this aspect of the program is not just to enable you to have a satisfying sex life but to help you reclaim the well-being and vitality that infuse your life with the creativity and energy that flow from a healthy sex drive.

HOW TO USE THIS BOOK

The Antidepressant Survival Program is an integrated approach in which the components work together to help you reclaim your vitality, sexuality, and desired weight. The program reflects the *medical* facts that

1. The various systems of your body and mind are intertwined.
2. Fixing a problem in one system will benefit the other systems.
3. If you don't solve a particular problem, it can have a domino effect, creating problems in other systems.
4. Addressing only one system rarely results in lasting health and well-being.

You may be tempted to skip around in the program, heading straight for the sex chapter, for instance, without incorporating the nutrition and exercise components into your life. But this would be a serious mistake, because you may well find that your sex life improves—without Viagra or hormone supplements—simply as a result of some healthy lifestyle changes. And, even more important, you will miss the significant and wide-ranging benefits of the rest of the program. A quick fix may take care of some of your problems for a while, but it will not help you achieve an energized and fit body and a full and vital life. To succeed at those goals you must think of your mind-body as a whole and work on all the systems together.

I realize that the thought of incorporating all the aspects of my program into your life at the same time can be daunting. In fact, I don't want you to. I've designed the program to phase in the various components at separate times so that you don't feel overwhelmed. I've created a time line, but you should feel free to move at your own pace, getting comfortable with one step and moving on *when you feel ready.*

I'd like you to begin with the Five-Day Jump Start, which I detail in Chapter 3. This is an eating and exercise plan with prescribed meals and activities designed to give you a firsthand experience of what your life can be like on my program. After just five days you will be motivated by the tangible results you've already achieved. After the Jump Start, you will want to *move directly* into the nutrition and exercise components of the program. It's important that you start altering your eating and exercise habits while you still have the momentum and motivation from the Jump Start. That's why I encourage you to familiarize yourself with the entire Fundamentals section of the program *before* you begin the Jump Start.

During these early weeks, I'd like you to visit your doctor and discuss the Antidepressant Survival Program with him or her. Take the quizzes in Chapters 8, 9, and 10, and discuss any symptoms you may be having with your doctor. Ask your doctor to consider the medical tests that seem appropriate for you and find out if you need to be referred to a specialist. (See Chapter 7 for specific advice on working with your doctor.) If you are a bit reluctant to talk this over with your physician, consider starting with your therapist, counselor, or even clergy. Work out a plan, and even consider having that person contact your doctor first, so that he or she is as receptive as possible.

After you've acclimated to the nutrition plan and exercise program—usually this takes about six weeks—you can begin to focus on relaxation techniques, getting play back into your life, and renewing your spirit. By this time your doctor should have obtained any test results and be ready to initiate the appropriate treatments.

To keep yourself on track, refer to this simplified time line.

Week 1	Weeks 2–6	Weeks 7–12	Weeks 13 and on
Jump Start (5 days)	Nutrition plan	Exercise program, Stage 2	Exercise program, Stage 3
Make a doctor's appointment	Exercise program, Stage 1	Spirituality plan (including play)	Maintenance of nutrition, spirituality
Find a "coach"	Initial doctor visit and testing	Second doctor visit and Medical Prescription plan	Maintenance doctor visits every 3 to 6 mos.

After guiding more than three hundred patients through the Antidepressant Survival Program, I have no doubt that it will work for you. The program is designed to give you a second chance at life. It will restore the healthful balance to your body, mind, and life that you may have lost—first as a result of your depression or other medical conditions, and then as a result of taking antidepressants. Once your balance is restored, you will feel rejuvenated and renewed—and your antidepressant medication will be working better than you ever imagined possible.

CHAPTER TWO

The Paradox of Antidepressants

How They Work Against Depression... and Sometimes Against You

* * *

*And it came to pass, when the evil spirit from
God was upon Saul, that David took a harp
and played with his hand: so Saul was refreshed,
and was well, and the evil spirit departed
from him.*

I SAMUEL 16:23

DURING MY PSYCHIATRIC TRAINING, the story of Saul came to mind in a new context. Even though he ruled as king over the biblical land of Israel, Saul was not satisfied with his life. He mistrusted his friends, isolated himself from his sons, and eventually committed suicide. He was given so much by God, yet he was never able to overcome his anguish. Saul was clearly suffering from a severe depressive disorder.

Depression has plagued humankind for at least as long as recorded history. Since biblical times those suffering from depression have turned to a host of remedies. Saul found solace in the music of David's harp. During the Middle Ages, when depression was thought to stem from spirits and demons, bloodletting and exorcism became popular forms of treatment. Beginning around the eighteenth century, the first mental hospitals or asylums were built to treat patients with depression and other mental disorders. Unfortunately, the "treatment" turned out to be more of a punishment; patients were shackled to the walls of their dark cells and visited only at feeding time.

It wasn't until the beginning of the twentieth century that depression was finally recognized as a problem worthy of medical attention. Sigmund Freud described depression as anger turned inward (a concept for which researchers have failed to discover significant evidence), and he used psychoanalysis to get his patients to talk through their problems. Freud's "talking cure" became a popular treatment for a variety of psychiatric problems, including depression. Freud's awareness that depression could also be the result of a *physiological* disorder didn't begin to take hold until the 1930s, with the advent of a new medical treatment—electroconvulsive therapy (ECT)—thought to restore moods by normalizing the brain's electrical signals. This invasive but highly effective antidepressant treatment (still useful in severely depressed, carefully selected patients) remained the medical therapy of choice until the first antidepressant medications came along, in the mid-1950s.

As is often the case with medical advances, one of the first antidepressants was discovered accidentally, when researchers testing a compound called iproniazid to treat tuberculosis noticed that the drug caused a pronounced elevation in mood in many patients. Iproniazid was a monoamine oxidase (MAO) inhibitor, a class of antidepressants that is still being prescribed today. Around the same time that MAO inhibitors came onto the market, researchers were testing another class of compounds with mood-elevating effects—the tricyclics. Tofranil became the first tricyclic antidepressant to be approved by the Food and Drug Administration in 1958.

By the early 1960s the floodgates had opened, and new treatments for depression began to pour in. Monoamine oxidase inhibitors and tricyclics came into widespread use. Then in the mid-1960s, neuroscientists announced a landmark finding: nerve cells in the brain communicated via chemical messengers—rather than via electrical signals, as had previously been believed. This discovery gave added credibility to the drug therapies being developed for depression. Depression would no longer be seen as a life sentence to be served out at a mental institution. It was a disease—just like cancer or heart disease—that could be, if not cured, at least managed with medication.

THE ANTIDEPRESSANT PARADOX

Antidepressants have offered hope and relief to millions of people suffering from depression and have saved tens of thousands of lives by preventing suicide. About two-thirds of people who are depressed will respond to any given antidepressant. Even if people don't respond to the first antidepressant they try, they will frequently respond to one with a different mode of action or to a combination of medications. What's more, antidepressants have proven effective at relieving a wide range of nondepressive disorders, including premenstrual syndrome, chronic pain syndromes, fibromyalgia, eating disorders, irritable bowel syndrome, migraines, chronic fatigue syndrome, and posttraumatic stress disorder—to name just a few.

Like all so-called magic bullets, however, most antidepressants have their drawbacks. They frequently cause side effects that leave people tired, woozy, and feeling like they're always "out of it." Other significant problems include weight gain; impotence; loss of sexual pleasure, desire, or orgasm; dry mouth; constipation; headaches; and gastrointestinal distress. Finally, antidepressants are not universally effective—only 60 to 70 percent of patients respond to even the most effective medications. Scientific literature classifies a successful response to antidepressant medication as a 50 percent or greater reduction of symptoms. *Thus, antidepressant medications actually can be said to relieve only 50 percent of the symptoms in 60 to 70 percent of patients.* A big help, yes. A stellar performance, no. The Antidepressant Survival Program is important because not only does it reduce or eliminate side effects, but it also makes your medication work more effectively.

Many patients find these side effects so difficult to deal with that they abandon their medications, only to see their depression recur. However, studies have found that people who have had one episode of depression have approximately a 50 percent chance of experiencing a recurrence if they stop taking antidepressants. Those who have had two or more episodes have an 80 percent or greater chance of experiencing a recurrence within a year if they stop their medications. Many, though, are not informed of this risk, or would rather take this risk than tolerate the side effects. What a terrible choice to have to make!

The trouble with antidepressants stems from their dual action in the body: they address the chemical imbalance that was caused by depression, chronic pain, or some other medical condition while disturbing the chemical equilibrium in other areas of the brain and body, ranging from the hormonal to the digestive system. Like the vast majority of medications doctors use, antidepressants cannot target only the problem they are meant to treat. They rebalance the activity of neurochemicals like norepinephrine, serotonin, and dopamine, and elevate moods by changing the receptor function of nerve cells—not only in the brain but throughout the body. This means that antidepressants can alter the workings of millions of cells from the brain down to the sex organs, which can impact the body's production of a wide variety of hormones and neurochemicals. The result: While rebalancing the body's mood-regulating neurochemicals, antidepressants create imbalances in many other important systems, which manifest as side effects.

TRICYCLICS AND MAO INHIBITORS: HOW THEY HELP AND HOW THEY HURT

Tricyclics, named for their three-ringed molecular structure, were the most commonly prescribed antidepressants for thirty years—until Prozac came onto the market in 1988. Tricyclics have a 60 to 70 percent success rate in alleviating depression, a rate that remains unsurpassed by any antidepressant medications, new or old. But many people who take tricyclics—such as Tofranil, Norpramin, Elavil, Pamelor, Vivactil, Surmontil, Sinequan, and Anafranil—are afflicted with severe side effects. We don't know for sure how antidepressants of any type work, but the leading theory is that they prevent nerve cells in the brain from reabsorbing, or reuptaking, neurotransmitters that regulate moods.

Dry mouth, one of the most common side effects of tricyclics, can lead to gum disease if oral hygiene is not excellent. Some people also experience dry eyes—making it difficult for them to wear contact lenses—and blurred vision, not to mention a dangerous effect in those with a certain type of glaucoma. Tricyclics can also affect heart function in a variety of ways that can, in the vulnerable person, prove very dangerous.

Tricyclics can also lower blood pressure, especially in older people, which can lead to dizziness when standing up or getting out of bed. Other side effects include constipation, difficulty urinating, fatigue, and sexual problems (impotence, loss of sex drive, inability to achieve orgasm). Perhaps the most troubling side effect is that many people feel as if they are floating through their days. This feeling of sedation causes drowsiness, difficulty concentrating, and an overall dulling of mental acuity. Another insidious side effect of tricyclics is weight gain—up to 20 percent of body weight.

Monoamine oxidase inhibitors—phenelzine (Nardil) and tranylcypramine (Parnate) being the most frequently prescribed—work by inhibiting the enzyme monoamine oxidase and raising the levels of mood-enhancing neurotransmitters. But like that of tricyclics, their usefulness is undermined by their often severe side effects, which can include rapid heartbeat, sedation, dizziness, insomnia, sexual problems (inability to maintain an erection, loss of sexual sensation), constipation, and agitation. Most important, MAO inhibitors can trigger a dangerous reaction if a person consumes aged cheeses or meats, or other foods containing high amounts of the amino acid tyramine. Normally, this amino acid gets broken down by the enzyme MAO. Since the antidepressant inhibits MAO, tyramine can increase to dangerous levels, triggering a rapid rise in blood pressure. This reaction may cause severe headaches, flushing, profuse perspiration, blurred vision, vomiting— even stroke and, rarely, death.

SSRIs: A NEW GENERATION OF BENEFITS AND SIDE EFFECTS

From the 1960s to the late 1980s, the development of antidepressants remained fairly stagnant. Every few years a new antidepressant would be introduced, but always with major accompanying side effects. Some medications were sedating while others were stimulating. None could treat the depression without causing side effects of one type or another.

Scientists spent twenty years developing and testing compounds that would block the reuptake of the mood-enhancing chemical sero-tonin and do very little else. Finally, they found a compound, labeled 82816, that selectively blocked the reuptake of serotonin into transmit-ting cells; it was fluoxetine, otherwise known as Prozac.

Prozac was the first of a new generation of antidepressants called SSRIs (selective serotonin reuptake inhibitors). These compounds work, we believe, by increasing the amount of serotonin in the nerve synapses. The therapeutic action of SSRIs bolstered the theory that depression is caused by poorly regulated serotonin activity in serotonin nerve cells; regulating this neurotransmitter helps nerve cells commu-nicate more efficiently and, thus, boosts mood. Selective serotonin reuptake inhibitors work by regulating the chemical voice of serotonin, one of the messengers sent from nerve cell to nerve cell. One nerve cell releases molecules of serotonin, which cross the synapse and fit like keys into the serotonin receptor locks on the surface of a neighboring nerve cell. At last count there were at least 14 known types of serotonin receptors, which are present not only in the brain but on a wide variety of cells throughout the body, including those in the intestines, blood cells, immune system, and sex organs. In fact, over 90 percent of the body's serotonin exists outside the brain (predominantly in the gas-trointestinal tract).

Selective serotonin reuptake inhibitors can affect any or all of the serotonin functions in the body. For instance, Prozac can cause an increase in serotonin, acting on the serotonin type 1D receptor. This can prevent migraine headaches, a welcome result. On the flip side, Prozac can also cause an increase in serotonin at the site of type 2 recep-tors, which can trigger a host of unwelcome side effects, such as sexual problems, agitation, and insomnia (while helping to treat obsessive-compulsive disorder and bulimia). Some of the newer non-SSRI med-ications, like Serzone or Remeron, were designed to fit into only one or two serotonin receptor types, thereby limiting side effects.

Whereas tricyclic antidepressants created biochemical hurricanes to blow out a candle, Prozac was thought to be a focused puff of air. It supposedly wreaked less havoc on the body while getting the same job done. Prozac has since been joined by other SSRIs, including Luvox, Zoloft, Paxil, and Celexa.

When Prozac came onto the market, it was hailed as a wonder drug that would cure depression without any of the troubling side effects caused by tricyclics and MAO inhibitors. Millions of prescriptions were written for Prozac, which became one of the most frequently prescribed drugs in the United States. But what it delivered was a mixed blessing. At first the developers of Prozac thought it had a very specific impact on brain serotonin levels—and, relative to tricyclics and MAOs, it did. But as my colleagues and I began prescribing Prozac, we quickly came to the conclusion that it was not side-effect free—far from it.

It's true that SSRIs work more specifically than tricyclics and MAO inhibitors, and they do cause fewer serious side effects. They can, however, still cause problems that severely affect quality of life. The incidence of these side effects is far greater than what was initially recognized by Prozac's manufacturer, Eli Lilly and Company, in the *Physicians' Desk Reference*. This means that some doctors who are not familiar with antidepressant side effects may not be taking their patients' complaints seriously. In the years since Prozac came onto the market, researchers have been documenting the various problems that SSRIs can cause.

SEXUAL PROBLEMS

Clinical data published in the *Physicians' Desk Reference* indicate that only 1.6 percent of patients on Prozac experienced decreased libido, and 1.9 percent experienced sexual dysfunction. But subsequent studies from independent researchers began to find that the incidence of sexual side effects was drastically higher. One physician reported in 1993 in the *Journal of Clinical Psychiatry* that out of sixty male patients on Prozac, 75 percent reported that they experienced difficulty ejaculating during sex or were unable to ejaculate. Lowering the dose helped ease the problems, and stopping the medication alleviated them. Selective serotonin reuptake inhibitors have also been found to cause sexual problems in women, ranging from a loss of sensation during sex to an inability to climax. As more research weighs in, the data indicate that at least half of patients can expect to experience some sort of sexual problem as a result of taking SSRIs.

Four newer SSRIs—Paxil, Zoloft, Celexa, and Luvox—also have a high rate of sexual side effects. In clinical trials of Paxil, nearly 13 percent of men had difficulty ejaculating, and 10 percent had other sexual problems, including impotence and an inability to achieve orgasm. Among women, nearly 2 percent reported difficulty achieving orgasm. In the Zoloft trials 16 percent of men and 2 percent of women had sexual problems. However, these data are likely to be grossly underestimated if the same discrepancies hold true for these drugs as they did for Prozac. Based on my own patients' experience, I think all the SSRIs cause approximately the same level of sexual dysfunction as Prozac does, although Paxil may be the worst offender.

Weight Gain

Despite the manufacturers' initial findings that Prozac and other SSRIs don't cause weight gain, researchers, clinicians, and patients have been indicating just the opposite. Research is still trickling in, but reports are indicating that people who take SSRIs for longer than three to six months frequently gain weight. This may explain the initial clinical data, which found that people lost weight during the first six weeks they were on SSRIs. In fact, Eli Lilly considered seeking approval of Prozac as a treatment for obesity based on its initial clinical trials.

Physicians were taken aback when they began to see weight gain in their patients on SSRIs. One researcher described the phenomenon as "completely unexpected" and stated, "We would be remiss if we do not inform our patients that weight gain may be associated with the use of fluoxetine [Prozac]." A study, published in the *International Clinics of Psychopharmacology,* found that 23 to 40 percent of psychiatric inpatients gained weight after two months of treatment with Prozac. Many of my patients have more intense carbohydrate cravings, probably the result of several mechanisms altered by the SRRIs. Others find that they simply gain weight more easily. Although more research is needed, I've found a definite link between weight gain and SSRIs in my patients.

Other Side Effects

Selective serotonin reuptake inhibitors can have varying effects on sleep, ranging from insomnia to hypersomnia (excessive need for sleep). Some SSRIs (Prozac, Zoloft) are more likely to cause insomnia, while others (Paxil, Celexa, Luvox) are more likely to cause hypersomnia, but because we are all wired a bit differently, the effects may be completely opposite in some people. For example, SSRIs may either alleviate or cause tension or migraine headaches. Prozac and Zoloft in particular can have a stimulant effect, causing agitation, nervousness, or anxiety in 10 to 15 percent of patients. An additional one in five patients on SSRIs (most commonly Paxil or Luvox) may feel drowsy or drugged. At least 5 percent of people stop taking their medication because of this side effect.

Since the vast majority of serotonin production in the body is related to the gastrointestinal tract, it is not surprising that all of the SSRIs can cause digestive disturbances, such as nausea and diarrhea. As an example, Prozac can cause nausea (in 21.1 percent of patients), diarrhea (12.3 percent), dry mouth (9.5 percent), indigestion (6.4 percent), abdominal pain (3.4 percent), and vomiting (2.4 percent). This class of drugs can also cause excessive sweating, skin rashes, abnormal dreams, and seizures (in about 0.2 percent of patients, which is about the average rate as far as most antidepressants go, with the exception of Wellbutrin—immediate release form, but not sustained release form—and Anafranil, which carry a higher risk, and Desyrel and Serzone, which do not increase seizure risk at all). Although SSRIs are much better tolerated than older antidepressants, it is clear that they're a far cry from side-effect-free miracle drugs.

CHANGING ANTIDEPRESSANTS TO ALLEVIATE SIDE EFFECTS

If you are experiencing troubling side effects from your antidepressant, your first course of action *could* be to try a different medication. Wellbutrin and Serzone, two of the newest antidepressants, have different side effects and a completely different mode of action from SSRIs, tricyclics, and MAO inhibitors. They aren't associated with weight gain or sexual problems. Like all medications, though, they are not without their side effects. Thirty-two percent of patients experience agitation, and 20 percent experience tremors while taking Wellbutrin. Serzone causes drowsiness in 25 percent of patients and can cause dry mouth, constipation, nausea, and dizziness, as well as have interactions with other drugs, such as Xanax.

Of course, you need to discuss with your doctor whether you could safely switch to a different medication. Two options you might explore are reducing your dosage or changing the timing of your dose. Studies have indicated, however, that dosage reduction may not be a safe alternative, since it appears that the dose that gets you well is the dose necessary to keep you well. I will only rarely consider dosage reduction as a reasonable alternative unless my patients have successfully integrated the Antidepressant Survival Program into their lives, thus lowering the risk of relapse. Changing the timing of your dose is a reasonable approach to reducing side effects such as drowsiness or even sexual dysfunction, which can both be worse when the level of medication is at its peak in your bloodstream.

If you have gone through several antidepressants and found that one is better at relieving your depression, you should probably stay on that medication and work on alleviating its side effects and increasing its benefits through my program. By the same token, you may need to be on a combination of antidepressants. (Many doctors, including myself, have found that combinations of agents actually work better than a single one, in some cases even canceling out side effects.) If you haven't yet tried switching medications, however, your doctor may be able to prescribe a different antidepressant that is just as effective but with fewer side effects.

Manipulating antidepressants requires expertise, which is why I strongly recommend that you see a psychopharmacologist if you decide to go this route. Most primary-care physicians (and even many psychiatrists) aren't well versed in the side effects caused by each antidepressant, and they may not understand the interactions among combinations. Psychiatrists who are certified in psychopharmacology by the American Society of Clinical Psychopharmacology (see Appendix One) have demonstrated expertise in prescribing antidepressants and other mood-altering medications. They also understand how these medications affect the body and are more familiar with their side effects. You can get the name of a psychopharmacologist in your area by contacting the American Society of Clinical Psychopharmacology at (212) 268-4260 for a referral. Keep in mind that the optimal goal is to find a medication that stabilizes your moods with a minimal number of side effects. You may not be able to find an antidepressant that is side effect–free, but you'll be able to find one that allows you to have a full life once you begin following my program.

A WORD ABOUT ST. JOHN'S WORT

St. John's wort has received widespread attention as a natural and effective way to treat depression. Sales of St. John's wort extracts have skyrocketed in recent years as more and more Americans self-medicate with this herb, which is available over the counter. The selling points of St. John's wort are that it is "natural," it causes fewer side effects than antidepressants, and it eliminates the need to work with a doctor while helping to reduce depressive moods. A spate of clinical trials conducted in Europe found that St. John's wort has antidepressant activity in mild to moderate cases of depression. It is not, however, a reliable substitute for antidepressants in people who are diagnosed with moderate to severe depression. Nor is it known to be effective for the myriad of nondepressive disorders that antidepressants treat.

I have a number of concerns about St. John's wort. My biggest is that it may cause toxic interactions if you're taking another antidepressant at the same time. I've had a number of patients come to me on an antidepressant and self-administered St. John's wort, unaware of the potential dangers. Researchers aren't exactly sure how the herb works. It may act like an MAO inhibitor, like an SSRI, or perhaps like both. Serious and even fatal reactions, including hypothermia and coma, have occurred when people have taken Prozac in combination with an MAO inhibitor. This means that if you're taking Prozac or some other SSRI, you could have a potentially serious reaction when you add St. John's wort to the mix, since there's a possibility that it has some MAO-inhibiting effects. The bottom line is that combining antidepressants and St. John's wort is uncharted and potentially dangerous territory.

Another concern I have is the unreliability of some companies that produce St. John's wort. I worry that depressed people who believe that St. John's wort is equivalent to other antidepressants might treat themselves unsuccessfully. If they use a brand that is low in quality—Kira is a reputable brand that I can recommend—they will not have a good response and may conclude that no treatment will work. Finally, it is important to understand that the fact that a substance is found in nature doesn't mean it is safe. Arsenic, for instance, is a natural element that is highly toxic in minute amounts. *Most important, the vast majority of the patients I see have multiple biochemical abnormalities that St. John's wort won't affect.*

A WORD ABOUT SAM-E

SAM-e (S-adenosylmethionine) is another nonprescription supplement that has been suggested to be useful in treating depression, fibromyalgia, and arthritis. Levels of this interesting substance, an amino acid derivative naturally found in the body, have been shown to be low in a significant number of depressed individuals. The level of SAM-e in the body can be increased by the use of intravenous SAM-e or oral antidepressant medications. Several well-designed double-blind, placebo-controlled studies indicate that SAM-e—*when administered intravenously*—may be an effective antidepressant medication, as well as useful in treating fibromyalgia.

There is currently no evidence that SAM-e works for the nondepressive conditions for which antidepressants are therapeutic, aside from fibromyalgia. Other unresolved issues in the clinical use of SAM-e include quality control and how well it can be absorbed when taken orally. Finally, for biochemical reasons, some patients may do poorly on SAM-e. Because of these unanswered questions, SAM-e cannot currently be recommended as a first-line treatment for moderate to severe depression, or for any of the other conditions that respond to antidepressant medication (aside from fibromyalgia, perhaps).

HOW MY PROGRAM CAN HELP
ELIMINATE SIDE EFFECTS

The Antidepressant Survival Program will increase the benefits of your antidepressants and relieve their most troubling side effects. My patients have found that the program has helped reduce their mental fog, sexual problems, memory lapses, sleep disturbances, weight gain, and gastrointestinal conditions. The program isn't able to alleviate every single side effect of antidepressants—for instance, it won't clear up a rash or dry mouth. But I can promise that you'll regain your lost vitality, youthful body proportions, mental alertness, and sexuality, which you need in order to fully regain your sense of self. Good sex may not be sufficient for a happy life and self-esteem, but it surely improves your chances.

I can also promise that you'll find yourself enjoying life more. You'll be enjoying the way your body looks and moves, and the innumerable pleasures that you have forgotten to make time for. You will also find, as your side effects recede, that your antidepressants are having *more* of a beneficial effect on your moods. This is the Antidepressant Survival Program at work, and it is a sign that the program is restoring the ideal neurochemical and hormonal balance in your body and mind, the equilibrium intended by nature. Once your balance is restored, you'll view life from an entirely new and poised perspective.

CHAPTER THREE

Getting Started

The Five-Day Jump Start

* * *

*Once begun, a task is easy;
half the work is done.*

HORACE, 8 B.C.E.

IF YOU'RE ON ANTIDEPRESSANTS you may well feel like a dead battery on a cold winter morning. No juice. Stalled out. But if you can hook your jumper cables up to a live battery—*zap!*—your engine kicks over and roars back to life. A jump start doesn't cure the underlying problem with your battery—you still need to drive to the shop and check under the hood—but it recharges you enough to get you rolling in the right direction.

Inertia is the enemy of change. And embarking on the Antidepressant Survival Program requires some major life changes—which can be overwhelming, even paralyzing. I begin my program with a Five-Day Jump Start because we all need a jolt of motivation to convert our passive, potential energy into active energy.

We resist change unless and until we grow so unhappy with our lives that we *must* change. But motivation—dissatisfaction with our current situation—isn't enough. We also need:

1. New ways of thinking about the problem
2. A plan for change
3. The energy to execute that plan and the commitment to succeed

Before my patients begin the program, we usually have some variation on the following dialogue.

Patient: I want to feel better. I need more energy and vitality in my life. What should I do?

Me: Are you willing to do what I tell you for five days? *Just five days?*

Patient: I don't know. What exactly do I have to do?

Me: You have to give up caffeine and alcohol, sweets and chocolate. You have to eat exactly what and when I tell you to, and exercise as instructed. You have to sleep seven to eight hours per day. Do this for only five days, and I promise you, you will be amazed at how you feel. Patients tell me they are amazed all the time. Do it and see if you feel better. If not, tear up the Jump Start and I'll never bother you with it again.

Patient: Can I just have one cup of coffee in the morning?

Me: No. You have to adhere to this plan religiously, without wavering, for five days. No coffee, no alcohol, no sweets. Only what is on the plan. You don't have to do it until you're ready. It will take some planning. Are you ready to commit?

Patient: OK, I'll try it.

Me: No. To try means to fail. It means you are telling yourself that if a good enough excuse happens to come up—and good excuses are never in short supply—you don't have to follow the plan. So you don't "try" it. Either you commit to it for five days or you don't. If you aren't ready to do it now, you can wait until you feel ready. When do you think you will be ready?

At this point my patients have to decide if they are ready or not to take the plunge. You have to face the same question.

ARE YOU READY TO BEGIN THE JUMP START?

You're the only one who can decide if you're ready to take action. The fact that you're reading this book is evidence that you've already taken the first steps. James Prochaska, Ph.D., a University of Rhode Island psychologist who has conducted research on how people alter their behavior, has found that remedial action is preceded by three stages:

Stage 1: Precontemplation. This is a state of automatic, nonthinking, or reflexive behavior. You feel that your situation is hopeless or you deny that you are experiencing a problem.

Stage 2: Contemplation. You accept that there is a problem and begin to *think seriously* about changing it. (This is probably where you are right now, seriously contemplating change.)

Stage 3: Preparation. You develop a firm, detailed plan of action.

The Five-Day Jump Start is the beginning of that detailed action plan. Read it over, and set aside a time when you can focus on how you're eating, exercising, and sleeping. You'll need some preparation—shopping for different foods or buying a new pair of walking shoes. Most important, you need to do the Jump Start at a time when you can make a 100 percent commitment. So think ahead about your obligations and deadlines. You don't want to do this program while trying to prepare your tax returns at the last minute or planning the final details of your child's wedding.

After all this ominous buildup, I want to reassure you that just about anyone can adapt to change for five days. Virtually all of my patients make it through this five-day program and walk away smiling. About 80 percent of them experience more energy and feel significantly better on the Five-Day Jump Start. Even more important, they are more likely to succeed on the Antidepressant Survival Program if they start with a manageable five-day commitment, which gives them a real feel for what the program can do.

Consider Joan, a forty-eight-year-old professor at a local university, who had been seeing me off and on for depression for six years. Although I had prescribed the antidepressant Paxil, Joan frequently fiddled with her dose, stopping and starting the prescription depending on how she felt. She complained that Paxil made her feel like she was floating through her days. She never felt completely alert when she was lecturing and frequently fell asleep while she was grading papers in the early evening. Joan was even more troubled by the fact that she had gained fifteen pounds since she had started back on Paxil several months earlier. She told me she constantly craved carbohydrates, like pretzels and chocolate chip cookies. "I keep a bag of each in my desk and constantly munch on them during office hours. I can't control it! But about an hour after eating them, I feel even more tired." Needing an energy boost to get through these troughs, she turned to coffee—at least four large mugs a day.

Not surprisingly, Joan was thinking again about going off the Paxil. I convinced her to try the Jump Start instead. "Give it a full five days and see how you feel," I told her. Joan followed all the meal plans, which, of course, meant cutting out pretzels, chocolate chip cookies, and coffee. When I met with her a week later, Joan recalled, "For the first three days, I had intense cravings for my chocolate chip cookies. I also felt tired and headachy from not having any coffee. But on the fourth day, I felt a little better. And by the last day, I could really feel an increase in my energy from where I used to be. I didn't feel like I needed my morning cup of coffee, and I stopped thinking about the chocolate chip cookies. I'm surprised at how much better I feel. How much more energy I have. And I'm much more patient with my children." Joan smiled. "They told me to thank you."

I explained to Joan that she had experienced a small taste of how she'd feel on my Antidepressant Survival Program. "If you can commit to eating the right kinds of foods, exercising, and making some overall lifestyle changes, you will feel even more energy than you do right now," I said. Joan was convinced, and she's been following my program for three years now.

During her most recent visit, I asked Joan what she felt she had gained from the program. "I understand now how much impact I can have on the way my body acts and feels," she told me. "I always thought that I was subject to every whim of my body, but now I realize that I can have a great deal of control over my energy and health."

Although it lasts less than a week, the Jump Start is a transforming experience. There's nothing so profoundly empowering as discovering we can become the masters of our bodies and minds. During the Jump Start, you'll be eating different kinds of foods and getting your body to move in ways it may not be used to. Your body will respond to these changes in lifestyle like a weak battery getting a jolt of energy.

A CHANCE TO RETHINK YOUR HABITS

The energy boost you get from the Jump Start will cause you to rethink the way you eat. Although my patients run the gamut from those who subsist on chocolate bars and fast-food burgers to those who count every gram of fat, 95 percent of them are filling their bodies with processed foods like breads, pasta, and packaged meals when I first see them. What's more, the vast majority of them have been eating way too many carbohydrates at the expense of enough protein. Does this sound familiar?

For five days I'm asking you to give up coffee (see Breaking Your Caffeine Addiction, page 59) and other foods that contain caffeine (yes, that includes chocolate), as well as foods containing refined sugar (cookies, cakes, pies, ice cream). And I'm asking you to abstain from drinking alcoholic beverages. Caffeine, sugar, and alcohol are the three biggest saboteurs of antidepressants. They wreak havoc on your moods, energy levels, and weight for reasons I'll explain in the next chapter.

Your initial reaction may be to view the Jump Start as a deprivation eating plan—and an unwelcome one at that. After all, there may be so few pleasures in your life, you probably don't want to give any of them up. While you may feel deprived for a few days, that feeling will quickly be replaced by the sensation of a "clean energy" boost, induced by giving your body the foods and exercise it needs instead of giving in to the cravings caused by the antidepressants. You're banishing the artificial energy boosters that surreptitiously rob you of your vitality in the long run. Instead, you're increasing your energy naturally through a well-balanced diet, exercise, and the proper amount of sleep.

Sleep is a very important part of the Jump Start. You need to get about eight hours a night to enable your body to replenish its energy (see Why You Need to Get Enough Sleep, page 60). In fact, many of my patients find that their sleep improves on the Jump Start. Charlene, a fifty-three-year-old patient of mine, was taking Prozac to control her anxiety attacks, but she found that the antidepressant wasn't able to alleviate her sleep problems. "I wake up every hour throughout the night," she told me. "I'm so exhausted during the day that I sometimes forget where I parked my car."

Charlene's eating habits were typical of most of my patients'. She drank about two cups of coffee a day and ate large servings of bread, pasta, and other starches with every meal. I told her that the combination of the caffeine stimulus (which can have pharmacological effects on brain and body chemistry for up to fifty-five hours) with the carbohydrates (which can cause blood-sugar dips during the night) was the likely source of her frequent sleep disruptions. "If you exercise, stop your caffeine, decrease all those processed carbohydrates, and increase your intake of protein, you'll probably be able to sleep more deeply," I told her. Charlene went on the Jump Start, and after four days she called me with great excitement. "I've slept through the night for the first time in fifteen years!" She felt encouraged to take the next step and begin the program.

The Jump Start is a day-by-day plan that maps out all your meals and gives you instructions for exercise. My intent in giving such detailed instructions is not to be rigid or authoritarian (in fact, you'll have choices between two meal plans and exercise routines). Rather, I've found that it's easier for my patients to follow the Jump Start if there aren't too many options to choose from. Once you get into the Fundamentals and Medical Prescription parts of the program, you'll have plenty of variety and choice.

In Chapters 4 and 5, I'll fill you in on the science behind the nutrition plan and exercise program. For now, let's just concentrate on the fact that you are taking charge of your body. Use the Jump Start as a way to focus and heighten your awareness of how directly food and exercise can affect your energy and mood—and alleviate the side effects of your medication.

I want to warn you that during the first few days you may feel headachy and drowsy. That's a sign that your body is withdrawing from caffeine, sugar, and alcohol (depending on which of these you currently indulge in). The severity of your reaction is an indicator of your physical dependency on these drugs. Even though you may not be feeling great, you're restoring your body to a healthier state. The majority of my patients are surprised to find that by day four they are feeling even better than when they started it. They notice that they have more energy (without their coffee or sugar fix), they feel relaxed in the evening (without their after-dinner cocktail), and they sleep better. Emotionally and physically, they feel like they're on a more even keel.

These feelings of well-being are your mind-body telling you that you're giving it what it wants. But the Jump Start is only a hint of what's to come. You won't enjoy the full benefits of the program until you master the Fundamentals and treat any hidden health problems outlined in my Medical Prescription.

The recipes and foods on the five-day eating plan can all be prepared in advance (or you can use the Quick and Easy Eating Plan that follows). Plan to spend some time on a Saturday or Sunday shopping for food and making some of the salads. (None of the recipes takes more than twenty minutes of preparation time.) When food shopping for the Jump Start, go to an organic supermarket whenever possible. Treat yourself to the best chemical-free produce and whole grains. You might need to pay a little more for these higher-quality foods, but you'll find the price is small compared with the benefits of better health.

READY, SET, GO!

If you have decided that you are ready, it's time to grab a calendar and set a start date for yourself—preferably within the next two weeks. Write down the foods you are going to buy, any new exercise gear you want (jump rope, shoes—keep it simple at this point), and the times and ways you plan to exercise on each of the five days. Figure out what you need to do and whose help you may need to enlist to ensure that you'll get a full eight hours of sleep for five nights.

Jump-Start Worksheet

Your Jump-Start Date _____

Shopping list:

_____

_____

_____

_____

_____

_____

Day, time, and type of exercise you plan

Day 1   (A.M./P.M.)   to   (A.M./P.M.)

Type of exercise _____

Day 2   (A.M./P.M.)   to   (A.M./P.M.)

Type of exercise _____

Day 3   (A.M./P.M.)   to   (A.M./P.M.)

Type of exercise _____

Day 4   (A.M./P.M.)   to   (A.M./P.M.)

Type of exercise _____

Day 5   (A.M./P.M.)   to   (A.M./P.M.)

Type of exercise _____

THE QUICK AND EASY EATING PLAN

Many of my patients tell me that they want a menu plan that's very simple and easy to follow—no special seasonings or ingredients or recipes. I give them this one-day plan of meals, with just enough variety to get through five days. If you prefer this plan, follow it every day for the entire Five-Day Jump Start. If you want larger portions, just keep the food ratios the same. (For example, if you want two sandwiches, make them both open faced, and increase your salad and fruit accordingly.) For a more varied menu of eating options, see the five-day eating plan that follows, which also offers vegetarian alternatives for meat dishes.

Note: If you have special medical conditions (such as migraines, cardiovascular disease, kidney disease, liver disease, or diabetes), show the Five-Day Jump Start plan to your doctor and make sure that it is safe for you. You may need to modify the plan under your doctor's supervision. *If you have an alcohol dependency, or if someone you know feels that you do, don't reduce your alcohol intake unless you are under medical supervision.* Sudden withdrawal from alcohol can cause tremors, hallucinations, agitation, and subtle brain damage in people who are alcohol-dependent.

If you are already an avid exerciser you will require somewhat less protein and somewhat more carbohydrate. Your meals and snacks should consist of less than one-third protein and more than one-third carbohydrate.

Breakfast

3 large egg whites and one large whole egg prepared any style*
1 medium orange
1 whole-wheat English muffin*
Water
*For vegetarian plan, use 2 teaspoons margarine to prepare eggs and eliminate the English muffin

Snack

$^1/_2$ cup plain nonfat yogurt topped with 1 tablespoon chopped peanuts and 1 tablespoon Grape Nuts cereal

Lunch

4 ounces canned albacore tuna (packed in water) with 2 tablespoons each green pepper and yellow onion and 1 tablespoon reduced fat mayonnaise
1 slice reduced fat Swiss cheese
or
4 ounces boneless, skinless chicken breast grilled in 1 teaspoon canola oil
$^1/_2$ cup cooked carrots
and
2 slices whole-grain bread
2 cups mixed greens salad with 1 tablespoon regular Italian dressing and 1 tablespoon pine nuts
1 cup blackberries
1 medium apple
Water

Vegetarian Option

1 cup vegetarian canned beans, mixed with 1 teaspoon Dijon mustard and 1 tablespoon barbecue sauce, sprinkled with 2 tablespoons reduced fat mozzarella cheese, and heated
1 slice whole-grain bread
2 cups mixed greens salad with 1 tablespoon of regular Italian dressing
1 cup blackberries
1 medium apple
Water

Dinner

4 ounces of baked or broiled fresh salmon or trout
or

4 ounces medium skinless, boneless chicken breast, baked or broiled
1 cup cooked broccoli topped with 1 tablespoon sunflower seeds
1 medium baked potato with skin with 1 tablespoon salsa
Water

Vegetarian Option

4-ounce veggie burger with 1 slice reduced fat Swiss cheese
1 cup cooked broccoli topped with 1 tablespoon sunflower seeds
1/2 medium baked potato with skin with 1 tablespoon salsa
Water

Snack

1/2 cup 1 percent milk-fat cottage cheese*
1/2 cup diced peaches
*For vegetarian plan, 1 cup 1 percent cottage cheese

Note: If you tend to get dizzy, irritable, headachy, or light-headed when you go without food for three or four hours (and if food alleviates the symptoms), you *must* have the snack between both breakfast and lunch, and lunch and dinner. *Everyone* must have the snack before bed. This will improve sleep and make it easier to wake up.

THE FIVE-DAY EATING PLAN

For people who want more variety, I have suggested different meals for each of the five days. You can interchange any of the main courses or side dishes, and you can increase the portion sizes. However, don't add extra fruit or starch without increasing the amount of protein you eat proportionately (unless you are very active physically). These meals are designed to give you a balance of protein to carbohydrates, so if you increase your carbohydrates you must also increase your protein. If you are not certain exactly how much protein (meat, fish, chicken, eggs, turkey, tofu) to eat, make your meal heavier in protein and lighter in carbohydrates (starches, fruits, and vegetables). I have also offered vegetarian options alongside the entrees that contain meat, chicken, or fish.

DAY ONE

Breakfast

Cheese omelet (4 large egg whites and 1 large whole egg, with 1 ounce shredded Muenster cheese, prepared in a nonstick pan sprayed with cooking spray.)
1 slice whole wheat toast with 2 teaspoons margarine*
1 medium pear
Water
*For vegetarian plan, eliminate toast and margarine

Snack

$\frac{1}{2}$ cup nonfat yogurt topped with 2 tablespoons chopped walnuts (1 tablespoon walnuts for vegetarian plan)

Lunch

Tuna melt (Mix 4 ounces water-packed tuna, 2 tablespoons chopped red pepper and 2 tablespoons regular Italian dressing; spread on one slice of whole-grain toast. Top with 1 slice reduced-fat American or provolone cheese; broil or microwave.)
2 cups mixed greens salad with 1 tablespoon of olive oil and balsamic vinegar to taste
1 medium orange
Water

Vegetarian Option

Baked eggplant slices (Cut 1 small eggplant lengthwise into $\frac{1}{4}$-inch-thick slices and arrange on baking sheet. Brush with 1 teaspoon olive oil. Top with 1 medium tomato, sliced, 5 ounces shredded, reduced-fat mozzarella cheese, $\frac{1}{8}$ teaspoon salt, and pepper to taste. Bake at 375° F for 15 minutes.)
2 cups mixed greens salad with 1 tablespoon of regular Italian dressing
1 medium orange
8 ounces skim milk
Water

Dinner

4 ounces skinless, boneless chicken breast
¾ cup cooked brown rice mixed with 2 tablespoons each broccoli, celery, and onion, 1 teaspoon minced garlic, and 1 teaspoon olive oil
½ cup steamed green beans with lemon juice
¼ cup dried fruit mixture (raisins, apricots, dates)
Water

Vegetarian Option

10 ounces low-fat firm tofu, cubed, marinated in 1 tablespoon reduced-sodium soy sauce and 1 teaspoon peanut oil. Stir fry with ½ cup cooked brown rice.
½ cup steamed green beans with lemon juice
¼ cup dried fruit mixture (raisins, apricots, dates)
Water

Snack

(I recommend a snack between meals and, if you have trouble sleeping, at bedtime. These snacks are optional and should be eaten when you feel hungry.)
1 cup combined sliced cucumbers and cherry tomatoes dipped in 2 tablespoons hummus
½ cup 1 percent milk-fat cottage cheese*
1 medium peach
*For vegetarian plan, ¾ cup 1 percent cottage cheese

Note: If you are lactose intolerant (have difficulty digesting dairy products), replace all dairy products with soy-based products, available at health and organic food stores.

DAY TWO
Breakfast

1 large hard-boiled egg
½ cup 1 percent milk-fat cottage cheese*

1 slice whole-wheat toast
2 teaspoons margarine
1 cup skim milk
17 grapes
Water
*For vegetarian plan, 1 cup 1 percent cottage cheese

Snack

5 reduced-fat whole-wheat crackers topped with 1 slice reduced-fat cheddar cheese

Lunch

Pasta salad (Combine 2 tablespoons each drained, cooked, or canned black beans and chickpeas, 3/4 cup pasta twists, 1 cup romaine lettuce, 1/2 cup shredded red cabbage, 2 tablespoons regular Italian dressing*)
1 cup strawberries
Water
*For vegetarian plan, 1 tablespoon regular Italian dressing

Dinner

6 ounces blackened tuna (Sprinkle with lemon juice and blackened-fish seasoning; broil until fish flakes.)
1/2 cup cooked brown rice with mushrooms
1/2 cup steamed zucchini
1 cup hearts of palm on dark green lettuce with 1 1/2 teaspoons vinaigrette dressing
1 1/4 cups watermelon cubes
Water

Vegetarian Option

Zucchini-mushroom casserole (Slice 1 large zucchini and sauté in 2 teaspoons olive oil for 2 minutes. Add 1/2 cup sliced mushrooms and cook for an additional 3 minutes. Remove from heat and stir in 4 beaten egg whites and 1 tablespoon shredded, reduced-fat moz-

zarella cheese. Season with salt, pepper, and garlic powder to taste.
Bake at 350° F for 30 minutes.)
1 cup cooked brown rice
1¼ cups watermelon cubes
Water

Snack

2 ounces reduced-fat feta cheese served on 1 slice pumpernickel
toast drizzled with 1 teaspoon olive oil and chopped fresh basil

DAY THREE

Breakfast

2 slices light whole-grain bread with 2 tablespoons light cream
cheese and 4 ounces lox*
2-inch wedge honeydew melon
1 cup skim milk
Water
*For vegetarian plan, replace cream cheese and lox with 2 ounces
reduced-fat cheddar cheese; have only 1 slice whole-grain bread

Lunch

Chicken salad sandwich (Mix 3 ounces boneless, skinless, diced
roast chicken, 2 tablespoons each celery and onion, 2 teaspoons
reduced-fat mayonnaise; serve on 2 slices whole-grain bread.)*
10 small green or black olives
½ cup cherry tomatoes
Fruit shake (In a blender combine ½ cup sliced strawberries,
½ medium sliced banana, 1¼ cups each skim milk and ice cubes;
puree until smooth.)

Vegetarian Option

Egg salad sandwich (Combine 2 large hard-boiled egg whites and
2 large whole hard-boiled eggs, 2 tablespoons each celery and
onion, and 2 teaspoons reduced-fat mayonnaise, served on 1 slice
whole-grain bread.)
10 small green or black olives

½ cup cherry tomatoes
Fruit shake (In a blender, combine ½ cup sliced strawberries, with 1¼ cups each skim milk and ice cubes; puree until smooth.)

Dinner

4 ounces London broil (Press ¼ teaspoon cracked black pepper into London broil; grill. Sauté 3 tablespoons minced onion and ½ cup chopped mushrooms in 1 teaspoon canola oil. Cook until onion is golden. Stir in ¼ cup low-sodium chicken broth and 1 tablespoon cornstarch. Stir until gravy is thickened and pour over meat.)
¾ cup roasted new potatoes
½ cup steamed snow peas with ½ teaspoon margarine
2 cups spinach salad with 1 tablespoon regular creamy dressing
1 medium pear
Water

Vegetarian Option

1½ cups low-fat cheese ravioli with ½ cup red pasta sauce, topped with ½ cup chickpeas sauteéd in 1 teaspoon olive oil
½ cup steamed snow peas with 1 teaspoon margarine
2 cups spinach salad with 1 tablespoon regular creamy dressing
Water

Snack

6 whole-wheat melba rounds with ¼ cup black bean spread*
*For vegetarian plan, replace melba rounds with ½ yellow bell pepper

Note: The Jump Start is designed to break your addiction to caffeine. This means no coffee, tea, chocolate, or caffeinated colas. Decaffeinated beverages are not allowed because they contain some caffeine, and they keep you one step closer to the real thing. If you are used to drinking coffee each day, you may experience symptoms of caffeine withdrawal while on the Jump Start. Another option is to wean yourself off caffeine slowly a week or two before you begin the Jump Start (see Breaking Your Caffeine Addiction, page 59).

DAY FOUR

Note: This day's menu is entirely vegetarian.

Breakfast

Egg on a muffin (Scramble 3 large egg whites and 1 large whole egg; place on whole-wheat English muffin with 2 teaspoons margarine, and top with 1 slice reduced-fat American cheese. Toast until cheese is melted.)
2-inch wedge cantaloupe
Water

Lunch

Curried millet-bean salad (Sauté ¼ cup each chopped onion and green bell pepper in 1½ teaspoons olive oil; sprinkle with ¼ teaspoon curry powder. Stir in ¼ cup canned kidney beans, ½ cup chickpeas, ⅔ cup cooked millet, ⅓ cup chopped plum tomato, and 1 tablespoon light sour cream. Chill before serving.)
1 medium orange
Water

Dinner

Spinach fettucine in cheese sauce (In food processor, puree ¾ cup fat-free ricotta cheese, ½ cup skim milk, 2 ounces shredded, reduced-fat mozzarella cheese, and 2 tablespoons grated Parmesan cheese. Pour mixture into nonstick skillet sprayed with cooking spray and add 5 ounces frozen, thawed chopped spinach. Stir over medium heat until heated through. Mix with 1 cup cooked egg-enriched fettuccine noodles.)
Water

Snack

Nachos (Spread 8 reduced-fat tortilla chips on a plate; top with ¼ cup canned black beans, 3 tablespoons salsa, and 3 tablespoons shredded, reduced-fat cheddar cheese. Heat in microwave until cheese is melted.)

DAY FIVE

Breakfast

1 cup 1 percent milk-fat cottage cheese
1 cup strawberries*
1 whole-wheat English muffin*
2 teaspoons margarine
Water
*For vegetarian plan, ½ cup strawberries and half a whole-wheat English muffin

Lunch

Turkey club sandwich (Combine 5 ounces sliced turkey breast, 3 slices tomato, 2 romaine lettuce leaves, and 1 teaspoon Dijon mustard and 1 tablespoon regular mayonnaise on 2 slices toasted whole-grain bread.)
½ cup red bell pepper drizzled with 1 teaspoon regular creamy salad dressing
1 cup pineapple chunks
Water

Vegetarian Option

Health sandwich (Melt 3 ounces reduced-fat cheddar cheese in 1 piece of whole-wheat pita bread. Stuff with ¼ cup chickpeas, ¼ cup cherry tomatoes, 2 tablespoons bean sprouts, 1 tablespoon sunflower seeds, and 1 teaspoon regular salad dressing.)
½ cup red bell pepper drizzled with 1 teaspoon regular creamy salad dressing
½ cup pineapple chunks
Water

Dinner

Lemon-ginger sole (Top 6-ounce sole fillet with 3 slices lemon and 1 teaspoon sliced gingerroot; drizzle with 1 tablespoon sesame oil and broil.)
1 cup cooked couscous with 1 tablespoon pine nuts

1 cup steamed green beans with balsamic vinegar to taste, pinch dill
2 apricots
Water

Vegetarian Option

4-ounce veggie burger topped with 1 slice reduced-fat provolone
cheese and ½ sliced green pepper
½ cup cooked couscous with 1 tablespoon pine nuts
1 cup steamed green beans with balsamic vinegar, pinch dill
Water

Snack

6 reduced-fat whole-wheat crackers topped with 1 tablespoon natural peanut butter
1 medium apple

THE FIVE-DAY EXERCISE PLAN

Of course, you won't get physically fit during the Five-Day Jump Start, but you will experience some of exercise's mood-boosting and body-enhancing effects. You'll also see how vital exercise is for increasing your energy. To reap the maximum benefits, you need to do a combination of steady (aerobic) activity and strength training. I explain the medical reasons for this in Chapter 5.

During the Jump Start, I'd like you to aim for twenty to twenty-five minutes a day of steady activity (walking, biking, jogging, and so on) plus fifteen minutes of strength training. You can break your activity up into ten-minute segments spaced through the day if you have a hard time finding a block of forty minutes.

I've outlined a five-day exercise plan. Feel free to do any of the activities on any days or do just one of the activities for all five days. If you're an avid jogger or tennis player, continue your favorite activity if that's your preference, but add the strength training. You might also consider using the Jump Start as a time to try adding something new to your exercise routine. As mentioned before, *make sure to plan ahead when you are going to exercise, what you are going to do, and where you are going to do it.*

Note: Clear this exercise plan with your doctor first. If you are not in good physical condition, start slowly, according to your physician's recommendations. Stop your exercise immediately if you feel any pain (chest pain, painful breathing, joint or muscle pain), and immediately consult with your doctor before moving forward.

DAY ONE

Aerobic Activity

Do a brisk twenty-minute power walk around your neighborhood or on a treadmill. (Make sure you have good walking shoes.) Power walking is done by taking short, quick strides and pumping your arms quickly to match your pace. Over the first five minutes, increase your speed until you are walking just slightly more slowly than a jog. You should find it somewhat difficult to carry on a conversation while walking at this speed.

Strength Training Move

1. Abdominal curls

Lie flat on the floor. Keep your knees bent and your arms across your chest. (You can cross your hands behind your neck if you need support, but don't use your arms to pull yourself up.) Rise slowly, looking at the ceiling, curling each vertebra separately until your shoulder blades are just off the floor, contracting your stomach muscles as you rise. This means your lower back should still be on the floor. Lower yourself slowly to work your abdominals even more.

Do 3 sets at 15 repetitions each, resting one to two minutes between.

2. Deep knee bends

Holding on to a chair back, do 3 sets of 10 repetitions each.

DAY TWO

Aerobic Activity

Use any piece of exercise equipment you have that gets your heart rate elevated. Dust off that stationary bike or bring out an old aerobics video. You can even buy a jump rope for five dollars and alternate one minute of jumping with five minutes of marching in place. You can walk up and down five flights of stairs in your office building, holding on to the rail. You can also buy a guest pass (for around ten dollars) to a health club and work out on a StairMaster, Lifecycle, treadmill, or rowing machine. Do this for twenty minutes.

Strength Training Move

1. Modified push-ups

Get on your hands and knees, with your hands shoulder-width apart, fingers pointing forward. Lift your calves off the floor, cross your ankles, and lower your torso toward the floor until your elbows are bent at a ninety-degree angle. (*Note:* Keep back and neck flat.) Then push straight up. Do 3 sets of 15 repetitions each (even if you have to rest between repetitions).

2. Shoulder press

Sit on a straight-backed chair holding two objects of equal but light weight (for instance, books, dumbbells), one in each hand. Raise both hands over your head, then return hands to shoulder height. Do 3 sets of 15 repetitions each, resting one to two minutes between sets.

DAY THREE
Repeat Day One.

DAY FOUR
Repeat Day Two.

DAY FIVE
Repeat Day One.

Breaking Your Caffeine Addiction

The Jump Start is the ideal time to break your addiction to caffeine, since you need to abstain from all caffeine in the nutrition plan outlined in Chapter 4. Unfortunately, studies have shown that people who need the caffeine equivalent of just one cup of coffee a day will experience symptoms of caffeine withdrawal if they miss their daily infusion. These symptoms include headaches, irritability, low energy, and fatigue, and can last up to four days. Symptoms of too much caffeine include diarrhea, irritability, insomnia, panic, palpitations and rapid heart rate, increased blood pressure, anxiety, and gradual weight gain.

You can avoid caffeine withdrawal, if you prefer, by slowly weaning yourself off caffeinated drinks (coffee and sodas) before beginning the Jump Start. Reduce your caffeine intake by 25 percent of your daily intake every two or three days. You should have your addiction broken within two weeks. If you feel headachy after you've reduced your intake, stay at that amount for an extra day or two before reducing your intake further.

You may decide to quit caffeine "cold turkey," which can cause caffeine withdrawal symptoms but has the advantage of helping you to understand that caffeine is as much a drug as any prescription medication. (I've often thought that if caffeine had to pass the Food and Drug Administration approval process, it would be labeled a controlled substance, since it is addictive, can reduce the seizure threshold, and can cause heart arrhythmias and trigger gastrointestinal distress.) If you choose this route, do it when the impact on your life will be minimal, such as on a weekend or during a slow period at work.

Remedies for caffeine headaches include a warm shower or bath, drinking at least eight 8-ounce glasses of water throughout the day, an over-the-counter pain reliever (make sure it doesn't contain caffeine), exercise, and time.

Patients often ask me: "How about decaf?" I prefer that you avoid decaf beverages because they do contain some caffeine, and because decaf keeps you one step closer to the real thing—and the temptation to relapse. Try out a few noncaffeinated herbal teas if you like a warm drink in the morning.

Why You Need to Get Enough Sleep

In order to restore your energy levels and sense of well-being on the Jump Start, you have to get the proper amount of sleep. Don't fool yourself into thinking that you need only five to six hours of sleep a night. Very few people can function well on that little sleep. Most adults need seven to eight and a half hours a night to achieve "optimal" rest, and some studies indicate shortening of the life span with less than normal amounts of sleep.

Researchers believe that sleep is a period of rest and recovery, restoring the brain and body after the physiological stresses of daily activity. Important hormonal and immune system activity happen during sleep. Getting too little sleep can impair your ability to concentrate, cause memory problems, and diminish your overall sense of well-being. So even if you follow all the other elements on the Jump Start, you may not feel an increase in energy if you aren't sleeping enough.

In recent years sleep researchers have begun focusing on the quality as well as the quantity of sleep. Good-quality sleep means that you go to bed drowsy, sleep deeply, and wake up refreshed. Here are some ways to improve your sleep quality:

* Use your bed only for sleeping and sex. Paying bills, balancing your checkbook, or doing work in bed will make you think of your bed as a stressful place. Doing these activities right before bedtime isn't a good idea either because they might make you too stressed to fall asleep.
* Take a short nap (if you need one) early in the day. Never nap after 2:00 P.M. or for longer than one hour. Taking long naps late in the day can depress your moods and make it very difficult to fall asleep at night.
* Avoid caffeine and alcohol. You'll be doing this anyway on the Jump Start. Although it's a depressant, alcohol interferes with sleep by disrupting sleep patterns, particularly in the second half of the night. You may fall asleep more easily, but you may wake up several times later in the night because you're sleeping more lightly or you have to urinate. A caffeinated beverage early in the morning will also likely affect your sleep at night. This may be hard to believe, since caffeine's effect seems to wear off within a few hours, but it's a fact.
* Keep a regular sleep schedule. Go to sleep and wake up around the same time each day. If you go to sleep late and sleep in on two consecutive days (over the weekend, for exam-

ple), you are unwittingly resetting your body's clock and may experience symptoms similar to jet lag.

* Don't exercise within three hours of bedtime. Exercise elevates your body temperature and quickens your pulse; this energy boost can last a few hours and make it harder for you to fall asleep.
* Keep your bedroom cool. Studies show that sleep is improved if the room temperature is on the low side (60 to 65 degrees Fahrenheit).
* Make sure you have a firm, comfortable mattress and pillow.
* Consider painting your bedroom a soothing color, such as a pastel (pink is known to be relaxing).

A PAT ON THE BACK FOR GRADUATES OF THE FIVE-DAY JUMP START

Congratulations! You've finished the Five-Day Jump Start. Riding out the energy lulls and food cravings that typically occur during the first three days of the Jump Start probably wasn't easy. Chances are excellent, though, that you began to feel better by the fourth and fifth days. You've begun to gain a sense of control over how you act and feel. You have taken hold of the reins and can now guide your body where you want it to go.

Your journey through the Antidepressant Survival Program is about to begin. The Fundamentals (described in the next three chapters) will continue the momentum of the Jump Start. *I urge you to begin this next part of the plan right after you finish the Jump Start, when your feelings of renewal and exhilaration are fresh.*

It's time to make a pact with the doubter who dwells within. Give yourself three months on the program—about the length of a season. That's enough time to become comfortable following the Fundamentals and to address any health problems in the Medical Prescription. If you don't feel better after three months, you can always go back to your old habits. The odds are stacked in your favor. If you are true to your three-month commitment, you'll notice such a dramatic improvement in how you feel that your internal doubter will join the cause.

The Fundamentals

Nutrition

* * *

Exercise

* * *

Spiritual Renewal

* * *

GOOD NUTRITION, EXERCISE, AND a renewed spirit are the keys to a fulfilling and healthy life. They are also fundamental to maximizing the benefits of antidepressant medications and reducing their side effects.

Think of nutrition, exercise, and spiritual renewal as the three legs of the stool that supports and sustains your wellness. If any one leg is unstable, the stool is likely to collapse. Working together, they create an efficient metabolism and a mind and body in balance. The more balanced you are, the better you'll feel—and the better you'll be able to absorb the destabilizing effects of antidepressants on your weight, your vitality, and your sexuality.

NUTRITION

Antidepressants require the right nutrients to enable them to do their job in your brain and body. Meanwhile, antidepressants can create unhealthy food cravings that lead to mood swings, energy depletion, and weight gain.

EXERCISE

In concert with good nutrition, exercise will normalize your brain-body functions in a myriad of ways. Exercise releases mood-elevating neurochemicals and circulates more oxygen to your brain, supporting the therapeutic action of antidepressants. When you're exercising regularly, you'll have more energy and your body can reclaim its youthful proportions. And by building your physical strength, you'll feel stronger and less vulnerable in both body and mind.

SPIRITUAL RENEWAL

Anyone who's recovering from depression or any other chronic ailment needs to take special care to nurture the spirit as well as the body. My prescription for spiritual renewal offers creative ways to restore your ability to experience pleasure by introducing stress relief, play, and spirituality into your life. If you're too stressed to enjoy yourself, you will never truly recover from depression. Play is an important ingredient in spiritual renewal because it increases access to pleasure by reinforcing dopamine pathways that may have become underactive during depression. And countless studies have affirmed the medical and psychological benefits of making some kind of spiritual practice—whether secular or religious—part of your daily routine.

The Fundamentals are the do-it-yourself part of my program, but please take note of places where I encourage you to enlist a coach or support person. Nutrition and exercise are areas you may want to explore in consultation with your physician, and a trainer or workout buddy can be an invaluable ally when you're trying to build exercise into your life. Spiritual pursuits are highly personal, but, again, the support of a community of people who share your beliefs or values can only increase the strength you draw from those wells.

CHAPTER FOUR

A Balanced Nutrition Plan

* * *

Let food be your medicine.

HIPPOCRATES

You've heard it a thousand times before. You are what you eat. Good nutrition provides essential high-quality fuel for the mind-body and is important for all aspects of your health. You're doubtless well aware that eating an abundance of fruits, vegetables, and whole grains (while avoiding saturated fats) can reduce your risk of heart disease and certain cancers. What you may not know is that these very same foods will also give you sustained energy and a general sense of well-being. What's more, eating the right kinds of foods can actually influence the workings of your genes and make you less susceptible to depression and other related illnesses.

Time and again you've experienced the intense effects that food can have on your moods. Cakes, cookies, and fudge are known as pleasure foods not only because they delight your taste buds but because they can make you feel calm and happy—at least temporarily. This sugar-induced sense of euphoria comes from several chemical mechanisms in your brain. First of all, the sheer pleasure of tasting a chocolate treat or powdery donut involves your brain's pleasure pathways and the release of dopamine and endorphins, the chemicals that make you feel

Auditing Your Eating Habits

Take this quiz to assess whether your eating habits could be contributing to your antidepressant side effects.

1. For breakfast do you eat starchy, highly processed foods (cereal, muffin, bagel, pancakes, donuts, or toast)?
   a. Yes   b. No

2. Do you regularly (once a week or more) eat any foods containing caffeine (coffee, tea, colas, chocolate)?
   a. Yes   b. No

3. Do you drink alcoholic beverages more than once a month?
   a. Yes   b. No

4. Do you regularly (once a week or more) consume high-carbohydrate snack foods (crackers, pretzels, baked chips, cookies, candy, soda, carrots)?
   a. Yes   b. No

5. Do you tend to have an energy slump about one to three hours after lunch?
   a. Yes   b. No

6. After dinner, do you graze through your kitchen, snacking on various foods?
   a. Yes   b. No

7. At mealtimes, do you eat . . .
   a. out of habit   b. because you're hungry

8. Do you eat more when you're stressed, anxious, bored, tense, or tired?
   a. Yes   b. No

9. Do you have protein (meat, chicken, fish, cheese, eggs) as the main course for lunch?
   a. No   b. Yes

10. Do you have protein as the main course for dinner?
    a. No   b. Yes

11. Do you crave chocolate or sweets frequently?
    a. Yes   b. No

12. Do you drink fruit juice on a regular basis (more than once a week)?
    a. Yes   b. No

Count your *a* answers and *b* answers. If you have four or more *a*'s, you need to reassess your eating habits and follow the plan outlined in this chapter.

---

exhilarated. You also get a quick surge of energy as the sugar hits your bloodstream. Unfortunately, that energized feeling lasts only as long as the sugar rush. Once your blood-sugar levels drop (about an hour or two later), you're left feeling drained and out of sorts. You become an addict looking for another hit.

Clearly, then, food can be as powerful as the most addictive drug. If you're experiencing carbohydrate cravings (independently or as a result of taking antidepressants), you're probably well aware of the addictive nature of certain foods. *Addictive foods are almost always processed foods.* (I have never known anyone addicted to lima beans.) And you probably know that feeding your cravings only makes you crave the food even more. In fact, some studies suggest that food cravings may be triggered by low levels of neurotransmitters (dopamine, serotonin, and endorphins), a phenomenon that may also occur in people who are addicted to alcohol and drugs. Research by Judith Wurtman, Ph.D., at the Massachusetts Institute of Technology found that women suffering from PMS-related mood swings felt calmer after eating carbohydrates;

carbohydrates help the body to absorb tryptophan, which can be made into mood-improving serotonin.

One of the first questions I ask my patients concerns diet. I ask them to tell me what they typically eat during the course of a day. Most of them wonder what their eating habits have to do with their state of mind or their use of antidepressants. They look at me in amazement when I tell them that their antidepressants can't work if they don't eat properly. Some of my patients are quite upset to learn that the antidepressants could be causing them to seek out certain foods to fulfill their cravings and get instant energy and that these very foods could be causing them to experience more severe side effects (weight gain, fatigue) and limiting the effectiveness of their medications.

In fact, most of my patients share similar eating patterns, and chances are you also follow these patterns. Here is a rundown of what they typically eat: For breakfast (many skip this meal entirely) they have juice, coffee, and a bowl of cereal, a muffin, or a bagel. Two hours later they feel hungry again, so they have another cup of coffee and a piece of fruit or some starchy snack, like pretzels. Lunch usually consists of a salad and sandwich with chips, washed down with a soft drink. About two hours later they experience a midafternoon slump and consume a sugary snack and a cup of coffee to get some energy. For dinner they pile their plates high with pasta, rice, mashed potatoes, or some other carbohydrate and may eat only a small amount of meat, chicken, or fish—if they have any protein at all. An hour or two after dinner, they feel hungry again and begin to graze on cookies, ice cream, and chips.

Most of my patients are dismayed to learn that the very foods they eat for energy, such as coffee and sugar, are leaving them more energy depleted. I tell them that they're listening to their addiction and antidepressants rather than their bodies. Antidepressants can trick your mind into thinking it needs sugar when you really need a well-balanced diet filled with protein, fruits, vegetables, and whole grains. And chances are you're not getting enough of these "medicinal" foods because you're filling up on "toxic" sweets. As a result, you may be deficient in protein as well as many key vitamins and minerals. And this sets you up for a double whammy: *Nutritional deficiencies can worsen the symptoms of depression and prevent a full recovery.* They can also increase vulnerability to the side effects of antidepressants, not to mention increased risk of a host of disorders, such as heart disease, cancer, and immune and hormonal problems.

Food can be either poison or nature's medicine. It depends on the types and sources of foods you choose to eat. All food is made up of macronutrients (protein, fats, and carbohydrates) and micronutrients (vitamins and minerals), as well as water and fiber. As your food gets broken down into its various nutrients, these molecules enter your bloodstream and are used to assemble chemicals and tissues within your body. Certain nutrients are used to manufacture neurotransmitters like dopamine, serotonin, and norepinephrine, which regulate your moods. Others bathe your cells and activate or deactivate certain genes that regulate everything from your appetite to your predilection for depression or other diseases.

For instance, your body uses the protein you eat, breaking it down into the amino acid L-tryptophan, the essential building block for the production of serotonin. Your body needs foods rich in zinc to manufacture testosterone, which fuels many brain-body functions besides your sex drive. Your body needs chromium-rich foods to help stabilize your blood sugar and mobilize your fat stores. Your body needs certain kinds of fats, called omega-3 fatty acids, found in cold-water fish, to help your nerve cells and immune system function normally. These are just a few of the many nutrients that will help lessen the side effects of antidepressants and will amplify the benefits of the medications, improving your mental health and your overall health as well.

In this chapter you'll find the tools you need to use food as a medicine rather than as a poison. If you're concerned about your weight, you'll find that you'll be able to lose weight without dieting by banishing your cravings for sweets and starchy snack foods. You will be eating the foods directly provided and intended by nature. Often I say to my patients, "If nature didn't grow it that way, don't eat it." (To make the point I ask, "Have you ever seen a bread, chocolate, or pizza tree?") *Choose foods that have been altered from their natural state as little as possible.* These are foods that are low in refined flours and high in fiber, that are low in processed sugar and high in whole grains, that are low in artificial ingredients and high in natural nutrients. Avoid preservatives, and, whenever possible, use organic foods, which are by definition grown without chemical pesticides, herbicides, fungicides, fertilizers, or hormones. Once you start to eat the foods that were intended by nature, you'll be restoring your body's natural balance of nutrients, and this will help restore balance to your body-mind.

I've given the eating plan outlined in this chapter to more than three hundred patients, and over 80 percent of them have experienced noticeable and surprising improvements in how they feel. You can expect to see these results:

* Your moods will improve, and you'll have fewer mood swings.
* The beneficial effects of your antidepressants will be amplified.
* Your energy will increase.
* You will lose weight or maintain a healthy weight.
* You may have an improved sex life.
* You will sleep better.

Realize that you are the one in charge. I can only write you a prescription for change. You will be the one to fill it, by fueling your body with the right kinds of foods. Accept the fact that you are in control of your body and that you make a conscious choice every time you put something into your mouth. But also realize that you will not be perfect; you'll improve your eating habits over time. Some people will adapt more quickly than others, but most important is the fact that you have chosen a new and healthier path.

MASTERING FOOD CRAVINGS

Although you are subject to intense food cravings, you must understand that you can make food choices that will significantly reduce or eliminate these cravings *before they strike*. You must also understand that when you crave a food, you may really be craving certain brain-body chemicals. In other words, your brain-body is so finely tuned that when it needs dopamine, endorphins, glucose, salt, or serotonin, it will guide you to those foods, chemicals, or situations that will provide a boost in those chemicals—even if those foods, chemicals, or situations have long-term negative effects. Your brain sends out a craving signal that it wants you to eat a particular food, and it wants you to eat it *now*!

You can prevent these cravings by keeping your brain-body chemistry in balance. In order to do this, you need to choose appropriate kinds of foods for meals and snacks. Rather than using a general multivitamin, *I prefer to target exactly what you personally need through the testing described in Chapters 8, 9, and 10.* Shortcomings of multivitamins are that they contain some elements that inhibit the absorption of other elements and that they are not targeted to your individual needs.

This eating plan will require you to make some major changes in the way you think about eating. If you're used to eating cereal for breakfast, a bagel for lunch, and pasta for dinner, you will have to plan some new meals. You will also be breaking your addiction to coffee and chocolate. In fact, that's the point of this eating plan: to break your addiction to foods that are known to be slow poisons. You may not feel great during the first two to seven days (depending on the strength of your addictions) after adopting this plan. (After all, you're going to be denying your body the foods that it craves the most.) But in a few weeks your body will have adjusted to your new eating habits, you will feel great, and you will continue improving. You'll have more energy, and you'll be more cheerful throughout the day. You will notice a subtle but amazing independence from your food cravings, and you will understand those people who can just stop eating when they are no longer hungry. You will also notice that your clothing is looser as you shed some of the weight you have gained on antidepressants.

GAINING HEALTH— NOT JUST LOSING WEIGHT

I want to emphasize, however, that *I'm not putting you on a weight-loss diet.* This program is a healthy foods diet. When used in conjunction with the other Fundamentals, it is designed to help you lose the fat (and pounds) you've gained as a result of your depression or of taking antidepressants. It will help you achieve and maintain the weight and body proportions that keep your body healthy.

You don't have to limit your portion sizes. You don't have to count calories or fat grams. You won't weigh yourself every week. (In fact, I don't even want you to use a scale.) You won't walk away from a meal feeling hungry or deprived. Your body will begin to crave a nutritious, well-balanced diet instead of cookies and crackers. You'll find that the pounds will come off naturally without your needing to make a conscious effort to lose weight.

Many of my patients who have gained weight on antidepressants ask: How quickly can I expect to lose weight? First, I remind them not to focus on weight. If they persist, I explain that the answer depends on how strictly they follow the Antidepressant Survival Program. People who follow the eating and exercise components of my plan usually lose about five to seven pounds during the first two weeks (much water weight). They then lose about a pound every week or two. Eventually their weight loss plateaus, and that means they've reached a healthy weight that their bodies are happy with. If not, they need to adjust other components of the plan.

It is preferable for the weight loss to be gradual, because this means you're adopting habits that you can live with for the rest of your life— not radical quick fixes that are likely to be temporary. Eating grapefruit or drinking liquid weight-loss shakes for breakfast, lunch, and dinner, besides being unhealthy, is not something anyone can do on a long-term basis. Eating natural, unprocessed foods in a healthy balance, though, is something humans have been doing for millions of years.

This nutrition plan is meant to be used in conjunction with the exercise program outlined in the next chapter. These two components go together to help you change your body—its proportions, weight, and muscle tone. On the nutrition plan you'll naturally eat fewer calories, and on the exercise program you'll be burning off more calories and reducing your appetite. The two components work together to help you strengthen muscle, which will boost your metabolism and help you return your body to its youthful proportions. (The relaxation-play plan outlined in Chapter 6 is the third key component that will help with weight loss by normalizing the stress hormones that may trigger your cravings for sweets and caffeine.)

Consider a patient of mine. Jan, a forty-one-year-old accountant, found that she had gained seventeen pounds over the two years she had been taking Prozac, which her family doctor had prescribed for her mood swings caused by PMS. "I became a bread addict," she said. She told me she ate a large bagel for breakfast, two or three scones from the bakery for lunch, and a large piece of buttered French bread with her dinner. She also complained that she still had mood swings. She usually felt somewhat calmer after eating but then felt moody in the late afternoon just before dinner. I told her about the program and explained the nutrition plan. "Given your high-carbohydrate, low-protein diet, your Prozac probably isn't working very effectively," I said. "And the more bread you eat, the more bread your body craves, and the more weight you gain."

The only solution was to break Jan's addiction. She followed my eating and exercise plan rigidly, in addition to the rest of the program, and found that her clothes were fitting more loosely after the first two weeks. She's now back to her regular dress size, and she told me she's amazed at how great she feels. She has more energy and no longer has mood swings. "The first week was pretty hard, because I craved bread all the time," she said. "But now I find that I've lost the cravings. I don't miss bread at all."

EATING FOR ENERGY

What convinced me that this nutrition plan works was, of course, the feedback from my patients. I myself was not much of a believer in the connection between food and moods until about a decade ago, when I saw a patient named Susan. I had been treating Susan for depression, posttraumatic stress syndrome, and chronic fatigue syndrome for about five years. We had tackled the first two conditions, but Susan continued to complain that she never had any energy. We tried one antidepressant after another, and although her moods improved she still had no energy. She told me her routine never wavered: Each day she came home from work as a bank teller at around 5:00 P.M. and crawled into bed. She had a part-time housekeeper who brought dinner up to her room and kept her house clean. On the weekends she would sleep most of the day. She told me she had no life.

Out of desperation I decided to test Susan for candida, an overgrowth of yeast in the intestines that has been claimed to cause multiple symptoms, including fatigue. I had read several books suggesting that yeast overgrowth can be at least partially caused by consuming too many refined carbohydrates. It turned out that she had an extremely high level of candida. When I questioned Susan about her diet, she told me about the chocolate cookies she would have as a morning snack at work, about the bagels she ate for lunch, and about the candy bars that kept her going in the afternoon.

I immediately instructed Susan to increase her intake of protein and to completely eliminate sweets (which are thought to promote the growth of yeast) and foods containing yeast, such as bread, mushrooms, orange juice, and beer. When I saw her a month later, she told me her housekeeper thought she had hired another housekeeper to help out. "I would go home, get into bed, and then realize that I wasn't tired! I had the energy to get out of bed, straighten the house, and make my own meals, so she figured I must have hired someone. The truth is, I was suddenly less tired and didn't need to be in bed in the early evening." I retested Susan for candida and found that her levels had been very much reduced.

I continue to see Susan for occasional therapy sessions, and she tells me that whenever she slips off the nutrition plan, she slips back into bed. While I cannot be sure whether it was the more well-balanced diet or the actual decrease in yeast (or a combination of the two) that brought back Susan's energy, I *can* say that her case made me a convert to the fact that food is an important variable in determining how well we feel in both body and mind.

This eating plan is designed as an ongoing lifestyle change. Since it requires you to eliminate certain foods from your life, you may, like Susan, fall off the wagon from time to time. But the problem is usually self-correcting. Having a pint of ice cream after dinner will make you feel lethargic and out of sorts in the morning. *Because of this time delay, most people do not make the connection between food and mind-body states.* When you do make the connection, you'll inevitably seek out those habits that will make you feel good again. Another helpful strategy to avoid slipping back for too long is to engage in this plan with a friend, or to ask your therapist to coach you.

After a while you will find that your once-favorite foods don't taste as good. In fact, most patients find that they lose their taste for high-fat sweets after they've gone off them for several weeks. So staying on this nutrition plan gets easier and easier. You just need to follow a few simple basics and aim for overall good eating habits. You will do it when *you are ready.*

THE THREE BASIC RULES

As I explained, I don't want you to count fat grams, calories, or portion sizes on this plan. Research has shown that people won't stick to complicated programs that require them to measure and analyze every morsel they put in their mouths. Get proteins and carbohydrates in the right combination, but don't count out every gram of protein and carbohydrate that you eat. Instead, follow these three basic rules.

Rule 1. At every meal and snack, eat balanced amounts of protein and carbohydrates. To do this, eyeball the portions on your plate. The carbohydrate serving should be a bit less than two-thirds of your meal (in volume), and the protein (which is more dense) should be a bit more than one-third (by volume). Use your energy as a gauge of which proportions are best for you. If you feel tired or hungry one to two hours after eating, you've probably overloaded on carbohydrates at the expense of protein, or you didn't listen to your feelings of fullness. You can get right back on track with your next meal.

Rule 2. Eat the least-processed foods. If nature doesn't grow it that way, don't eat it. As I mentioned earlier, this nutrition plan is based on foods intended by nature. Limit your intake of anything that contains flour or other refined carbohydrates. Choose whole-grain carbohydrates and fresh fruits and vegetables instead. Barley and lentils have far more natural nutrients than pasta and white rice. These foods are also less likely to cause unstable blood sugar, which means they won't leave you depleted of energy. Whenever possible, eat only organic foods, to reduce your exposure to neurotoxic pesticides and hormones.

Rule 3. Eliminate the four toxic foods: sugar, white (refined) flour, caffeine, and alcohol.

Commit to following these three rules for six weeks. Follow this nutrition plan *to the letter,* cutting out all the toxic foods while increasing your intake of the medicinal foods. After six weeks think about the foods you miss the most and—if you must—allow yourself small amounts of your favorite foods on no more than a once-weekly basis, always balancing the protein and carbohydrates as directed. The danger, of course, is a slow and subtle relapse into your old eating habits. *So if you allow yourself dessert once a week, keep it at once a week.*

Be wary of this strategy, though. If you have a serious addiction, even one dessert could lead to an uncontrolled intake of toxic foods. This could set you off course for weeks, months, or years (as in Jim's case; see page 92). Use your moods and energy levels as a gauge. (Lethargy and moodiness are your body's ways of letting you know that you've eaten too many toxic foods.)

THE TOXIC FOODS

The toxic foods are foods that you're going to have to eliminate or eat only sparingly because they are slow-acting poisons, adversely affecting moods, energy levels, and overall sense of well-being. They also cause you to pack on pounds, especially if you're taking antidepressants. What's more, they can interfere with the beneficial effects of your antidepressants.

SUGAR

If you're on antidepressants, sugar is the thing you crave most. It's also the very thing that will rob you of your energy and sense of well-being. Eating foods high in sugar activates an energy-draining cycle. Let's say you have a bowl of Frosted Flakes or a fruit Danish for breakfast. This high-sugar meal will cause your body to overproduce the hormone insulin, which helps your cells use the high amount of sugar that has entered your bloodstream. Repetitive high insulin levels reduce your body's ability to recognize the insulin; therefore, your cells can't use the sugar, so it is stored as fat. The insulin itself increases your hunger for carbohydrates—as well as your cortisol levels. You begin to crave a midmorning donut and/or coffee to give you some energy. Before you know it, you've gained weight. Even worse, you're too frequently tired all the time, feeling out of sorts, and always seeking food to give you more energy. You find yourself eating out of tiredness and anxiety, not real hunger.

Not everyone has such a negative response to sweets, but most antidepressants can leave you more susceptible by triggering intense carbohydrate cravings, which set you on the vicious insulin cycle. Paradoxically, the more you feed your cravings, the stronger the cravings will become. Scientists still haven't mapped out the exact mechanism for how antidepressants trigger sugar cravings. It probably has to do with the fact that these drugs affect the appetite centers in the hypothalamus, as well as their long-term effects on certain serotonin receptors.

My prescription for sugar: Elimination of sugar-filled foods from your diet is the only way to banish your cravings for good. After six weeks on the nutrition plan, limit your intake to one serving of dessert each week, and make sure you eat these foods with adequate amounts of protein. I'll tell you how to do this later in the chapter.

If you're trying to lose fat or improve energy and mental clarity, you must avoid sugar-filled foods altogether. Also, check food labels for hidden sugars such as glucose, maltodextrin, corn syrup, cornstarch, and modified cornstarch. Foods that are sweetened with honey or fruit juice are also no-nos. They can contain the same amount of sugar as or even more sugar than products that have the real thing.

CAFFEINE

Every time you have a cup of java or a Coke, the caffeine triggers a release of the hormone adrenaline, which, among other actions, signals the liver to release sugar into your bloodstream. You get a burst of instant energy from the sugar and adrenaline. But it lasts only two or three hours before you crash. That little energy boost can leave you feeling drained over the long haul. The result? You crave candy bars and cookies, the very foods you're supposed to avoid, to get more quick energy.

Caffeine is highly addictive, and it causes instabilities in your blood sugar, which raise your risk of obesity, diabetes, panic attacks, and even seizures (if you are prone to them). What's more, caffeine stays in your system for about two days, which means it can interfere with the quality of your sleep (which leaves you feeling tired, which causes you to crave caffeine and sugar, and so on). I've also found that some of my patients use caffeine as a substitute for exercise. They figure: Why do a workout if I can get a little boost of energy without the time and effort?

My prescription for caffeine: Eliminate all foods and beverages that contain caffeine. These include coffee, tea, caffeinated soft drinks, chocolate, and some pain relievers. See Breaking Your Caffeine Addiction on page 59 for information on weaning yourself off caffeine.

ALCOHOL

If you're feeling drained of energy, still experiencing symptoms of depression, or having sexual problems, the last thing you need is a depressant chemical. Yet that's what alcohol is, a chemical that slows down brain function and interferes with normal sleep. One study found that depression was a problem in 70 percent of people who had prolonged heavy drinking habits. I remember working with a patient whose depression didn't clear up with therapy and a series of medication trials. After a year on antidepressants, she finally told me that she was drinking heavily with friends on the weekends. I counseled her to stop drinking as an experiment and restarted the first medication we had tried. Within one month she had a complete response to her antidepressant.

Alcohol can also play a major role in weight gain, since it is a hidden source of calories. A glass of wine or bottle of beer contains about 150 calories. Some frozen tropical mixed drinks can have 300 calories or more. And alcohol will increase your appetite, encouraging you to eat more than you normally would.

Alcohol can be especially damaging if you're having sexual problems. Although alcohol can help you lose your inhibitions, its effects on the body are, for the most part, far from sexy. As blood-alcohol levels increase, penile blood flow decreases. Drinking also decreases vaginal lubrication, lengthens the time it takes to achieve orgasm, and weakens a climax's intensity. As alcohol dulls nerve pathways to leave you "feeling no pain," it takes its toll on other parts of the body as well, reducing sensation in the genitals and making foreplay less stimulating.

Often patients respond to my minilecture on alcohol with a legitimate question: "Doesn't alcohol have a protective effect on the cardiovascular system? Shouldn't I have a glass of red wine each day?" My answer is: "Do you want a healthy heart and an unhealthy brain?

Besides, there are many other ways—like exercise and a diet low in saturated fat—to have a healthy cardiovascular system that will help both your heart and your brain."

My prescription for alcohol: Avoid all alcoholic beverages (beer, wine, mixed drinks, cordials, and so on). Many of my patients tell me they are surprised by the greater clarity in their thinking, improved sleep, and enhanced energy and sexual function that come from abstaining from alcohol. You can try some nonalcoholic substitutes like seltzer with a twist of lime or a splash of cranberry juice. Or you can try nonalcoholic beers, although some of these products are high in sugar. (Read the labels carefully to make sure there's less than 8 grams of sugar per serving, and, of course, balance with protein.)

You will be surprised to notice that you can stimulate an artificial "high" just by holding and sipping a nonalcoholic drink in a setting where you usually drink alcohol, such as a bar or nightclub. This phenomenon, called conditioned learning, is well documented. Studies have shown that drug addicts who go through a withdrawal syndrome in a particular place, such as the street corner where they regularly bought their fix, will reexperience the withdrawal symptoms if they go back to that same street corner months after being drug free.

REFINED CARBOHYDRATES

The low-fat, high-carbohydrate diet that became so popular in the 1990s is nutritional suicide for someone taking antidepressants. Living on pasta, bagels, and bread can intensify your cravings for sweets and can leave you as lethargic as would a diet of chocolate éclairs and Oreos. It's no wonder most people find themselves gaining weight on these diets.

As you're probably beginning to suspect, not all carbohydrates are created equal. While it's true that your body breaks down all carbohydrates (whether from a pear, a pretzel, or a cookie) into glucose, the rate at which your body absorbs and breaks down carbohydrates varies tremendously depending on the type of food. Those foods that are broken down more quickly by the body are considered to have a high glycemic index. They enter the bloodstream quickly, raise blood-sugar levels rapidly, and are more likely to produce an exaggerated insulin response. Blood-sugar levels quickly plunge, and the body goes out of balance, leaving you tired and drained. Of course, high-sugar foods, like cakes and cookies, have a high glycemic index, which means they are rapid inducers of insulin. But so are cornflakes, pasta, instant mashed potatoes, most breads, and, of course, candy, sodas, and other sweets. (See Appendix Two for a complete glycemic index.)

This is probably because the more refined or processed a carbohydrate is, the more its molecular structure has been broken into small particles. These small particles are more easily absorbed and broken down by the body into glucose, which causes a surge in blood-sugar levels, excess insulin release, and so on. So eating pasta for lunch can trigger a midafternoon slump, which then triggers a craving for caffeine or sugar. Is this energy-depleting cycle starting to sound familiar?

Carbohydrates that are less processed and higher in fiber, like whole oatmeal, barley, and pears, are digested more slowly and produce more gradual elevations in blood-sugar levels. Certain exceptions are fruits and vegetables that are naturally high in the sugar fructose, such as bananas, raisins, corn, and possibly carrots, which may also have a high glycemic index.

My prescription for refined carbohydrates: Eliminate pasta, bread, white rice, crackers, pretzels, and other products that contain flour, cornstarch, cornmeal, milled corn, or other refined carbohydrates. Switch to natural whole grains, like barley, bulgur, and whole-grain rice. If you find it hard to live without pasta and bread, eat pasta made from whole-grain wheat and breads made from whole-grain wheat, pumpernickel, and rye. These have lower glycemic indexes than white breads and more processed pasta. *If you're trying to lose weight, cut out bread and pasta entirely, since they will sabotage your weight-loss efforts.*

I also recommend limiting your intake of certain fruits and vegetables that have a high glycemic index (see Appendix Two for a complete glycemic index of carbohydrates). Once you've reached healthy weight and body proportions, and feel a sustained increased amount of energy, you can add a once-weekly serving of refined carbohydrates back into your diet, always balanced with protein. But use your energy level as a cue: If you feel exhausted or moody after a meal, or the next morning, you need to reduce your intake of these foods.

CIGARETTE SMOKING

Cigarettes are, of course, toxic substances, and smoking can prevent you from getting your body into balance. Cigarettes cause breathing difficulties and hinder your ability to exercise; tar is also a culprit in smoking-induced lung cancer and emphysema. In addition, cigarettes can worsen the side effects of antidepressants: Nicotine constricts blood vessels, which can disrupt the blood flow to the sex organs and thereby aggravate any sexual problems brought on by antidepressants. It can also stimulate the adrenal glands to release stress hormones, which can aggravate an adrenal gland dysfunction brought on by a previous depression or medical condition.

Unfortunately, smoking appeals to people who are depressed. A survey conducted by the National Institute of Mental Health found that 76 percent of people with a history of depression "had ever smoked" compared with 52 percent of the general population. This is because nicotine acts in many ways like an antidepressant: It revs up your body and has a mood-boosting effect. Since smoking can also be difficult to stop, I don't recommend that you try to kick the habit while you're getting started on this program. Focus on incorporating the Fundamentals into your life, and give yourself a few months to get used to these lifestyle changes. Once you feel like your program has become a routine part of your life, you will be ready and able to tackle your smoking habit.

My prescription for quitting smoking: There are a number of options available when you're ready to quit smoking, but you will notice that quitting is easier once you have integrated the program into your life. First, your doctor may prescribe bupropion (called Wellbutrin or Zyban) to carefully add to your antidepressant regimen. Research has shown that bupropion counteracts nicotine withdrawal symptoms (headaches, fatigue, the jitters) and helps substitute for the antidepressant effects you get from cigarettes. Stay on bupropion for as long as your doctor advises.

Nicotine replacement therapy (available via a patch, chewing gum, and nasal spray), which delivers small, controlled doses of nicotine, is another option and has a 20 to a 45 percent success rate. I prefer the patch or spray to the gum because the dosage is more carefully controlled by those delivery systems. Scheduling is a method that involves a five-week behavioral program designed to gradually wean you off cigarettes. You can try any or a combination of these options.

You can also quit cold turkey, but I don't recommend this method, since it is the most physically and psychologically trying; you'll experience nicotine withdrawal symptoms almost immediately, and they'll last an average of three weeks. Your adrenal system will have to readjust to the absence of nicotine, and this can take a month or longer. Tapering slowly, or using a patch, allows this process to occur in stages.

THE MEDICINAL FOODS
PROTEIN

Your body breaks down the protein you eat into twenty-three amino acids. Eight of these are the so-called essential amino acids, which must come from diet via protein-rich foods. *Studies have repeatedly demonstrated that people on antidepressants who abstain from eating protein—even for as little as three days—will suffer a relapse of depression.* When they add protein back into their diets, they again respond to the antidepressants, in about three days.

Your body breaks protein down into amino acids. Tryptophan, one of the essential amino acids, is the core building block of serotonin, one of the neurotransmitters necessary for mood control and appetite suppression. Your body also needs protein to produce the pleasure-inducing neurotransmitters, dopamine and norepinephrine. If your body can't manufacture sufficient levels of these three neurotransmitters, your antidepressants won't provide their full benefits. My patients are frequently amazed at how much better their medications work once they begin to eat more protein.

It would be logical to wonder, after reading the preceding paragraphs, why not eat a diet of only protein? There are a multitude of reasons why this is unhealthy, but here are the three biggest ones: First of all, your body can handle only so much protein before your kidneys become strained, which can cause them to malfunction. Second, your body is better able to absorb tryptophan in the presence of carbohydrates (and the absence of certain other amino acids)—an interesting example of how nature loves balance. Last, protein alone won't give you sustained energy or keep your blood-sugar levels even. You need to eat protein in combination with carbohydrates and fats to get its full energy and mood-boosting benefits.

To understand why, let's get into a little science: If you were to eat a burrito filled with vegetables, cheese, and shredded beef, your body would use the various nutrients from your meal for blood-sugar control in a specific order. Within a few minutes to an hour after eating, the tortilla and vegetables (which are mostly composed of carbohydrates) will be broken down into glucose (a simple sugar), which will enter your bloodstream, causing your blood-sugar levels to rise and then fall again about an hour later. At that point the protein from the cheese and beef will have been converted to glucose and will again trigger a rise in your blood sugar. Just as your levels are about to fall once again, the fat from the cheese and beef will finally have been converted to glucose to trigger a third rise in your blood sugar. This total process takes about five hours—ending just in time for your next meal. So eating the right combination of carbohydrates, protein, and fat can keep your blood-sugar levels on an even keel to prevent energy lags and sugar cravings—which can help you lose weight.

My prescription for protein: The trick is to get the right ratio of carbohydrates to protein. Follow the two-thirds rule: Make sure the volume of protein is a little more than one-third of your meal (unless you are already an active exerciser, in which case your protein should be just under one-third of your meal), while carbohydrates are a little less than two-thirds. (Remember to count fruits and vegetables, in addition to starches, such as potatoes and grain-based foods, as carbohydrates.) So if you're having chicken and vegetable stir-fry for dinner, just under one-third of your plate should be whole-grain rice, just under one-third should be vegetables, and just over one-third should be the chicken. I recommend you stick with low-fat protein sources, such as fish (salmon, albacore tuna, herring, sardines), skinless white-meat turkey and chicken, extralean select grades of beef and pork (beef eye of round, top round, and top sirloin, and pork tenderloin), and low-fat vegetable protein (beans, tofu) for reasons that I'll describe in the next section.

If you're trying to determine serving size, the best rule of thumb is to eat a portion of beef, chicken, or fish that's about the size of a deck of cards. The total carbohydrates can cover two decks of cards. You can increase your serving sizes to reach your level of satisfaction of real hunger, but make sure you increase the protein by about the same proportion as you increase carbohydrates. If you are already exercising a good amount, do not increase the protein as much.

The rule of thumb to remember is that *you must always eat carbohydrates with protein.* Thus, a piece of fruit is an inadequate snack unless it's combined with a protein, like a piece of cheese, cottage cheese, or some turkey. Err on the side of eating a little extra protein (again, unless you are already an avid exerciser) rather than a little less. (If you have liver or kidney problems, consult with your doctor about how much protein to eat.) I'll say it again. Listen to your body: If you're feeling tired or drowsy after a meal or snack, you know you've eaten too many carbohydrates.

Omega-3 Fatty Acids — the "Good" Fats

Fat has become such a villain that I consider it the forgotten nutrient. Fat serves as a barrier to slow the entry of carbohydrates into the bloodstream. Fat also makes food taste better. Enjoying a satisfying meal stimulates your dopamine pathways, which temporarily improves your state of mind. Last, eating some fat can actually aid in reaching and maintaining a healthy weight, since fats help to satisfy appetite quickly. The fat and protein content in a meal causes the release of a hormone called cholecystokinin from the stomach. This hormone, among others, tells the brain you're satisfied and to stop eating.

Of course, you need to be selective about the kinds of fats you eat. The fats we get too much of in our modern Western diet are arachidonic acid and saturated fats (those that harden at room temperature). These fats are found in shellfish, egg yolks, dairy products, organ meats (like liver and most deli meats), and fatty red meats. Saturated fats are difficult for the body to process and help narrow arteries. I recommend you eat low-fat sources of animal protein.

Build your meals around the "good" fats. These are the monounsaturated fats and omega-3 essential fatty acids. Monounsaturated fats help reduce the risk of narrowed arteries, thereby improving your circulation, which can help keep your energy levels up, the flow of blood to your brain healthy, and your sex organs functioning properly. These fats are found in fish, olive oil, canola oil, flaxseed oil, olives, macadamia nuts, and avocados.

Omega-3 essential fatty acids can help make your nerve cells more responsive to chemical signals from serotonin, dopamine, and norepinephrine. A clinical trial conducted at Harvard University—reported in the September 1998 NIH workshop on omega-3 essential fatty acids and psychiatric disorders—found that manic-depressive patients who took fish oil capsules high in omega-3 fatty acids in combination with medication showed significantly greater mood stabilization. Epidemiologists have found that people who live in countries with seafood-based diets rich in omega-3 essential fatty acids have a significantly lower incidence of a number of psychiatric disorders, including depression and manic-depression, as well as other health conditions, such as heart disease (which is also closely associated with depression) and certain cancers. Moreover, recent studies have shown that depressed patients have much lower levels of these fatty acids than the normal population. Omega-3 essential fatty acids are predominantly found in dark-fleshed fish, including salmon, albacore tuna, mackerel, anchovies, caviar, herring, sardines, lake trout, and Atlantic sturgeon.

My prescription for fat: Eat at least one omega-3-rich fish meal a day—preferably two. Cook with canola and olive oil instead of butter, margarine, or vegetable oil. When making eggs with olive oil instead of butter, heat the oil to a high temperature before putting the eggs in the pan. Use flaxseed oil (another source of omega-3 essential fatty acids) or canola oil to make salad dressing, and baste olive oil on chicken or fish. Limit your intake of foods containing "bad" saturated fats and arachidonic acid, listed in the previous section.

FOLIC-ACID AND VITAMIN-B-RICH FOODS

In the 1960s a noted psychiatrist noticed that after consuming a diet deficient in folic acid for a few months, he developed fatigue, irritability, sleep disturbances, and memory problems. Since then there has been increasing evidence that you're more likely to feel depressed or remain in a state of clinical depression if your diet is deficient in folic acid, or vitamins B_6 and B_{12}. Your brain needs these B vitamins to initiate many essential chemical reactions that help prevent depression and heighten the effects of antidepressants. Studies have revealed that people who are depressed have significantly lower amounts of folic acid in their red blood cells. What's more, you don't need to be extremely deficient to suffer ill effects: It takes only a mild deficiency in these vitamins to fog your mind and reduce your concentration. (Abnormal gastrointestinal function, which I will review in Chapter 9, can easily affect the availability of B vitamins.)

Recently, I began treating a seventy-three-year-old man, Max, for low vitamin B_{12} levels. A successful businessman, he'd been feeling overwhelmed by life for two years—more and more depressed, to the point of feeling he couldn't go on. This occurred despite being on Prozac, which he had earlier responded to well. His blood tests for B_{12}-related abnormalities were on the borderline, so Max and I decided to give him a trial of B_{12} injections with folic acid—despite the disagreement of his internist. Max's response was so dramatic—his depression lifted and his energy doubled—that within three weeks we began discussing cutting back on therapy sessions.

The good news is that correcting these deficiencies can help to dispel any lingering depression and improve your concentration and memory. You'll be improving other factors of your health as well. Mothers who eat adequate amounts of this vitamin early in pregnancy are much less likely to have babies with spinal cord defects. Folic acid also plays a role in preventing heart disease (which is associated with depression) by reducing excess levels of homocysteine, which is believed to contribute to the damage of blood vessel walls. There is a weaker but still significant link between a shortage of vitamins B_6 and B_{12} and increased homocysteine levels. Vitamin B_6 also plays a role in easing the symptoms of PMS, which can involve mood swings, anxiety, sugar cravings, and feelings of depression. Are you beginning to see how huge an impact you can have on your mind-body through the foods you eat?

My prescription for folic acid and vitamins B_6 and B_{12}: Following my protein prescription for eating more meat, chicken, or fish will enable you to get adequate amounts of vitamin B_{12}—unless you have the kind of absorption problem discussed in Chapter 9. Protein-rich foods also contain (though in smaller amounts) vitamin B_6. Other vitamin B_6 sources include bananas and avocados. Folate-rich foods include all legumes, dark green leafy vegetables, Brussels sprouts, spinach, oranges, sunflower seeds, wheat germ, and peanuts. Aim for at least three servings a day of folate-rich foods: For instance, eating 1 cup of steamed lentils and 1 cup of spinach sprinkled with sunflower seeds will go a long way toward fulfilling your daily folate requirement. If you decide to supplement your diet with a particular B vitamin, always add in a complete B complex, such as Solgar B-Complex "50," so that you don't create deficiencies in any of the others.

CARBOHYDRATES INTENDED BY NATURE

As I mentioned earlier in this chapter, my nutrition plan is based on eating foods in their natural state. Unrefined carbohydrates (whole grains, fresh fruits and vegetables, legumes) offer major health benefits over processed carbohydrates. First of all, they are generally high in fiber, which improves digestion and controls the release of sugar into your bloodstream. Fiber may also help reduce cancer risk, improve cholesterol levels, and stimulate the growth of healthy bacteria in the digestive system. (Those bacteria manufacture several of the B vitamins you need for normal brain function.)

Another significant health benefit is that unrefined carbohydrates contain significantly more natural vitamins (like folic acid, vitamins B_6 and B_{12}) as well as minerals. For instance, nuts and whole-wheat grains contain zinc, which plays a major role in memory and mood control and is necessary for testosterone production. Calcium, plentiful in kelp, collard leaves, and turnip leaves, is necessary for the proper functioning of the dopamine pathways. Magnesium, found in dark greens, wheat bran, buckwheat, and rye, has numerous bodily functions, including the generation of energy from food.

I'd estimate that 90 percent of my patients taking antidepressants are somewhat deficient in one or more minerals, and chances are you are as well, especially if you're not eating a well-balanced diet. *One way to maximize your intake of minerals is to buy foods that are organically grown without chemicals, the way nature intended.* Research suggests that organically grown foods have a higher content of minerals because the soil that they're grown in is less likely to be depleted, since organic farmers can't rely on artificial fertilizers, pesticides, and herbicides to make the plants grow well in the absence of good soil. A recent study by Consumers Union, publisher of *Consumer Reports,* found unsafe, although not illegal, levels of toxic chemical contamination (including some nerve agents that are directly toxic to nerve cells) in peaches, winter squash, apples, pears, spinach, grapes, lettuce, celery, and green beans.

My prescription for carbohydrates intended by nature: Choose whole grains, fruits, and vegetables over refined, processed carbohydrates. Buy organically grown produce whenever possible.

SAMPLE MEAL PLANS

Here is a list of meal choices that have the appropriate proportions of carbohydrates to protein. The list should give you some ideas about the kinds of meals you can plan. But by all means go beyond this list, and aim for variety. The options for nutritious meals are endless.

Try to drink water, preferably bottled or purified, with meals. If you have juice, realize that it is a high-sugar carbohydrate that needs to be balanced with protein.

Breakfast

1. Slow-cooked oatmeal with a serving of cottage cheese
2. Vegetable omelet and a piece of fruit
3. Scrambled eggs (one whole egg plus three egg whites, or egg whites or Egg Beaters only) and one piece whole-grain toast (for those who want to keep food preparation simple and quick, the eggs can even be microwaved in less than two minutes—while your toaster is toasting!)
4. Whole-grain English muffin topped with a good serving of lox and a bit of cream cheese

Lunch

1. Open-faced tuna sandwich on a single slice of whole-grain bread
2. Three-bean salad (kidney beans, green beans, and chickpeas mixed with olive oil and cider vinegar)

3. Tofu and vegetable stir-fry
4. Grilled chicken salad (grilled chicken breast in mixed greens salad topped with low-fat dressing; ask for a double serving of the chicken)
5. Vegetarian burger topped with one slice cheese and served on half a whole-grain roll or one slice of whole-grain rye bread

Dinner

1. Broiled salmon or tuna steak (sprinkled with your favorite spices, such as garlic powder, lemon pepper seasoning, and olive oil) with green beans and barley
2. Chicken stir-fry (sautéed chicken breast cut into strips in sesame oil and soy sauce; add red pepper, scallions, fresh ginger, and water chestnuts)
3. Turkey burger (three-quarters of a pound ground turkey mixed with chopped onion, garlic, pinch of oregano, and black pepper; sauté in olive oil until brown; serve with baked beans)
4. Beef with broccoli (sauté beef and chopped garlic in sesame oil; add broccoli and cook until bright green; serve over small portion of whole-grain rice)

Snacks (calcium-rich)

1. One-half cup cottage cheese with fruit (see the Five-Day Eating Plan, page 49).
2. One-half cup plain or vanilla yogurt (see the Five-Day Eating Plan, page 49).
3. One cup of soy milk fortified with calcium and a rye cracker spread with peanut butter
4. One cup of skim milk and a rye cracker spread with peanut butter

KEEP A FOOD DIARY

Although you don't need to count every calorie or carbohydrate gram, you'll find that keeping track of what you're eating is a powerful aid, especially during your first six weeks on the nutrition plan, when you're still getting used to the new concepts. Moreover, it's too easy to

Daily Meal Record

Breakfast

Protein source _____ Estimated % of meal _____

Carbohydrate source _____ Estimated % of meal _____

Fluid _____

How you felt (mood, energy, and hunger)
90 minutes after breakfast: _____

Morning snack

Protein source _____ Estimated % of meal _____

Carbohydrate source _____ Estimated % of meal _____

Fluid _____

How you felt (mood, energy, and hunger)
30 minutes later: _____

Lunch

Protein source _____ Estimated % of meal _____

Carbohydrate source _____ Estimated % of meal _____

Fluid _____

How you felt (mood, energy, and hunger)
1 to 3 hours after lunch: _____

Afternoon snack

Protein source _____ Estimated % of meal _____

Carbohydrate source _____ Estimated % of meal _____

Fluid _____

How you felt (mood, energy, and hunger)
30 minutes later: _____

Dinner

Protein source_____ Estimated % of meal_____

Carbohydrate source_____ Estimated % of meal_____

Fluid _____

How you felt (mood, energy, and hunger)
90 minutes after dinner: _____

After-dinner or Bedtime snack

Protein source_____ Estimated % of meal_____

Carbohydrate source_____ Estimated % of meal_____

Fluid _____

How you slept, and how you felt (mood, energy, and hunger)
upon waking: _____

slide back into your old eating habits if you aren't monitoring yourself. Keeping a diary will help you stay conscious of whether you're getting enough protein and veering away from refined carbohydrates. You should also keep track of the tactics you use to incorporate the nutrition plan into your life. One rule of thumb I tell my patients: Shop the periphery of the supermarket (which has the produce and protein-rich meats, cheese, and fish) rather than the inner aisles (which tend to have more processed foods). Try this and record the results in your diary. You'll have a record to look back on if you slip off the plan.

Make a copy of the Daily Meal Record, and use it every day to fill in what you've eaten for your meals and snacks. Since your routine will probably vary, you need to think about your day's activities. Are you going out to dinner? Will you be on the road tomorrow during lunchtime? What lunch and snacks are you going to pack? Are you having guests for the weekend? How can you make your food choices interesting and healthy? Do you need to meet a client at a restaurant for breakfast? If so, what will you order?

Be honest with yourself! Record what you've eaten. This includes that cookie you sneaked from the pantry or that handful of jelly beans you grabbed from a co-worker's candy dish. All those nibbles can add up to an enormous amount of carbohydrates that you may not be accounting for. (They can very likely also be the culprit behind your still-sagging energy levels.) I would also like you to keep track of any symptoms (tiredness, low energy, irritability, mood swings, and so on) you may have felt through the day.

STICKING TO THE NUTRITION PLAN— WITHOUT CHEATING

I need to warn you that once you begin to feel better on my nutrition plan and have achieved a healthy weight, you may be tempted to let the rules slide. If you've ever been on a diet, you know how easy it is to go back to your old eating habits once you've achieved your desired weight—or even as you begin to notice a change in your weight. And you know how it starts: You allow yourself a bowl of ice cream after dinner, then you sneak a slice of birthday cake at a co-worker's party. Pretty soon you're eating more carbohydrates than ever, maybe without even realizing that you've gone back to your old habits.

This is exactly what happened to a patient of mine. Jim, a fifty-seven-year-old lawyer and father of two, came to me three years ago concerned that he had gained fifty pounds after he started taking Elavil (amitriptyline), a tricyclic antidepressant, for depression. Jim told me he ate a pint of Cherry Garcia ice cream every night after dinner. He also had two or three beers every day after work and a glass of wine with dinner. Jim came to me at his wife's urging. "She says I'm breathing too hard when I walk up the stairs in our house," he said. "She's terrified that my heart is a ticking time bomb that's waiting to destroy our lives."

I told Jim that his wife could be right. "My advice," I said, "is to say good-bye to ice cream and alcohol and say hello to exercise." We talked at length about how, when, where, and why, and Jim joined a health club and began lifting weights and walking on the treadmill. He exchanged his pasta salads at lunch for grilled open-faced chicken breast sandwiches. Instead of eating a donut during his coffee break, he grabbed some cottage cheese. Instead of eating pizza for dinner, he had a salmon steak with broccoli and a bean salad. Within six weeks Jim had lost four inches around his waist. He told me that he felt terrific and that he didn't feel hungry on his new eating plan. He said he couldn't believe how much of an energy drain his old eating and drinking habits were. Jim followed my eating plan pretty religiously for about a year. Then I lost track of him for about two years until his wife, Donna, came to see me.

"I'm really scared," Donna said. "Jim has totally gone back to his old ways. He's stopped exercising, and he's gained back all the weight." He had even embraced his two former loves: Cherry Garcia and beer. "Jim is too embarrassed to come see you because he doesn't want you to think he failed," she said. I convinced her to insist that Jim come in. When Jim came to see me, I asked him what had happened. "I was really into the plan and had lost all the weight I needed to, so I began to relax a little. I figured, 'OK, I've got this down,'" he said. "First, I just had a small bowl of ice cream, but pretty soon I was back to a pint a night. *The truth is, I wasn't even aware that I had gone off the plan.* It wasn't really a conscious choice. I just sort of slid off of it."

Jim had a strong family history of depression and heart disease, two diseases that have been linked to the American diet. (Alzheimer's disease, which is linked to inflammation of certain brain cells, is also linked to diet.) I explained the connections to him and convinced him to approach the plan not as a weight-loss diet but as a lifestyle change. Otherwise he was heading for serious trouble. Jim went back on the plan, and he lost three belt sizes in a month. But more than that, he told me he has a new awareness about the benefits he gets from eating the right foods. "I can really see the difference more clearly between my life on the plan and my life off of it."

I've found that a relapse is not such a bad thing. It gives people self-awareness and helps them put their lives into perspective. If you've been on the plan long enough to feel more energy, going off the plan will make you sluggish. When you restart it, you will realize much more clearly how much you gain by going back on it again. Of course I'm not telling you to go back to your old eating habits, but if you do, don't beat yourself up about it. Simply remember that you were able to get your life back once and you can do it again.

You can take heart from a recent study of eight hundred successful dieters who maintained an average weight loss of thirty pounds for five years or longer. The study found that the dieters needed several tries before they could commit to lifelong changes in their eating habits. It is important to figure out how and when you slipped off the plan (stress, sleep deprivation, overwork, and loneliness are major culprits), and how you will get back on it again. Think of your relapse and return to the program as a learning process, a way to reinforce to yourself that you are the true master of your body and that, as Hippocrates said, food *can* be your medicine.

Rethinking Dessert

"No more dessert? How am I ever going to follow this plan?" you might ask. It's true, many people live for dessert (for all those reasons previously discussed), and I'm not asking you to forgo all desserts. I'm asking you to rethink the concept of dessert. In fact, do up dessert like the French. They choose to dine on the sweetness and juices of a luscious peach complemented with cheese. The cream puffs and chocolate croissants are just for tourists! Here are some excellent dessert choices:

* Apple and cheddar cheese slices
* Trail mix of sunflower seeds, walnuts, and raisins
* Fresh blueberries mixed in cottage cheese or yogurt topped with wheat germ or granola
* Pineapple slices sprinkled with nutmeg, cloves, and cinnamon, and a handful of cashews
* Frozen strawberries blended with milk

If you must indulge

All of us want a rich dessert once in a while. But to keep your body in a state of vibrant health, you need to avoid these indulgences whenever possible. If you do have them on rare occasions, however, *be sure to balance them with adequate protein.* Also, plan ahead whenever possible: If you plan to have a dessert, reduce the carbohydrates in your main meal. For instance, forgo a serving of rice and eat extra chicken to compensate for the dessert at the end of the meal. If you suddenly splurge on a sugary treat, balance it with a few slices of turkey or cheese. (You may be eating some additional calories over the short term, but by helping to prevent mood swings and sugar lows, you'll be avoiding extra calories over the long term.)

COMMON QUESTIONS ASKED BY MY PATIENTS

I've noticed that cereal is not on the nutrition plan. Is it not allowed?

Breakfast cereal is a concentrated form of carbohydrates and often contains a lot of sugar. In fact, many nutritionists consider sugar cereals to be the nutritional equivalent of candy, and even the high-fiber bran cereals can be sugar-coated. Even brands that are low in sugar can have a whopping 49 grams of carbohydrates per three-quarter-cup serving. You would need to eat a four-to-six-egg omelet for every serving of cereal just to add the right balance of protein—and this doesn't include the carbohydrates in the piece of fruit or fresh juice you might have with the meal. Slow-cooked oatmeal is a much better breakfast choice. It enters the bloodstream more slowly and will give you more nutritional bang for your buck.

I've heard that high-protein diets can cause ketosis. Do I need to worry about this?

First of all, my nutrition plan is not a high-protein diet. It's just getting you the right balance of protein to carbohydrates. The plan will not put you into ketosis, but it will help you to lose excess pounds. Ketones are the chemicals made when your intake of carbohydrates is too low and/or your protein intake is too high. In this situation your body's stores of protein and fat are converted into an alternative fuel to glucose, called ketones. When ketones accumulate in excess, they can reduce your brain's use of oxygen, which can cause you to feel tired and a little woozy. Your body has to get rid of the ketones via urine, stool, and breath (causing an unpleasant odor or funny taste in your mouth). To avoid this, you must consume balanced amounts of carbohydrates and protein.

How quickly can I expect to lose weight?

This plan is designed for fitness and for regaining your youthful body proportions, but on it you will lose weight gradually. If you're following the exercise plan outlined in the next chapter as well as the nutrition plan, you can expect to lose around one pound per week. You might lose five to ten pounds during the first two weeks, but some of this is probably excess water that your body was retaining on a high-carbohydrate diet. Eventually, your weight loss will plateau, which may mean you will need to increase your activity levels to give your metabolism a boost (or adjust other aspects of the program). See Chapter 5 for details on the exercise plan.

Can I use artificial sweeteners instead of sugar?

My own preference is that you limit your intake of artificial sweeteners. They are reported to cause fatigue and irritability, and they could sabotage your efforts to banish your sugar cravings by feeding your sweet tooth. If you were previously eating a lot of sweets, your taste buds may be resistant to the stimulation of sugar, requiring more and more sweets to give you the pleasant sensation you desire. As you cut out the sweets, your taste buds will readjust, so you can eat smaller amounts of sweets to get the same taste sensation. You will probably be surprised when the sweets you once loved actually taste too sweet. You may find that you actually don't miss the sugary soft drinks or sugar cereals. But if you still need a sweetener in your diet, use *small* amounts of unrefined honey, maple syrup, or sugar.

Is fruit juice allowed on the plan?

I recommend only freshly squeezed juices, but even these contain little of the fiber and pectin found in whole fruit, which are sources of vitamins and other disease-fighting molecules called phytochemicals. Store-bought juices are so processed that they are often no better than sugar water. Many fruit "drinks" sold in supermarkets contain only 10 percent juice; the rest is water and various types of sugar and other sweeteners. If you like juices, I strongly recommend you consider buying a juicer. Although the process is time-consuming, you can mix fruit and vegetable juices and get highly concentrated amounts of vitamins and minerals from freshly squeezed juices. As an example, one glass of carrot juice can contain the beta carotene of ten to fifteen carrots. Fresh juice (vegetable and fruit) can be very nutritious as long as it is balanced with protein.

Where can I get recipes that have the right protein-carbohydrate combinations?

I have not included recipes in this book, but several other books contain recipes with the right protein-carbohydrate ratios. I recommend *Zone Perfect Meals in Minutes* by Barry Sears (HarperCollins, 1997). Recipes in this book are easy to follow, but some are heavy in breads and other refined carbohydrates. I would substitute whole grains, lentils, and beans for the breads wherever possible or at least use whole-grain breads and corn instead of flour (for instance, tortillas for the Mexican recipes). Another good book is *Protein Power* by Michael R. Eades, M.D., and Mary Dan Eades, M.D. (Bantam Books, 1996). It has interesting and nutritious recipes, although some contain alcohol and may be too high in protein, which you should adjust for. This book also includes a section on dessert recipes, but many of these call for artificial sweeteners, which you don't want to get hooked on. See Recommended Resources for other suggestions.

SUMMING UP

The nutrition plan encompasses two basic strategies.

* First, balance your protein with your carbohydrate intake so that protein provides roughly one-third of your daily calories and carbohydrates the other two-thirds. The fats will take care of themselves.

* Second, be selective about the proteins, fats, and carbohydrates you eat, always aiming for the most nutritious options based on a diet intended by nature.

You may need to avoid certain foods that your body is sensitive to or take certain vitamin or mineral supplements for nutrients you're deficient in. I'll discuss a personalized approach to your eating plan in Chapter 9.

Now, let's move on to the exercise program. You'll see that exercise goes hand in hand with the right eating habits to restore your vitality, boost your mood, improve your sex life, bolster the effects of antidepressants, and, of course, help you get to a healthy weight and youthful body proportions.

You're on the road to getting a life that's in balance, and you'll soon start to see how all the elements in my program are integrated and build on one another synergistically to enhance the beneficial results. *By following the entire program,* you will begin to regain the energy, motivation, and self-esteem that were missing from your life. You will recapture that joy you felt when you were young and dreaming about the life that lay ahead for you. You'll reexperience the freedom and hope that vanished when you became depressed. You'll finally be able to say, "I have a life, and I want to *live* it." You should always keep that goal in mind, even if you don't yet believe it's possible. You'll believe, once you feel it for yourself.

Remember that you are the architect of your life.

CHAPTER FIVE

A Balanced Exercise Program

* * *

*Those who think they have no time for
bodily exercise will sooner or later
have to find time for illness.*

EDWARD STANLEY

IF YOU'VE EVER GONE for a walk around the block to gain some perspective on an emotional crisis, you know just how important movement can be to improving your mood. Problems that seemed
overwhelming when you were standing still become easier to sort
through as you pound the pavement. Movement eases negative emotion, gives you self-awareness, *and* enables you to mobilize your mental
energy.

Study after study provides strong evidence that exercise plays a
major role in lifting mood. An analysis of eighty studies found that
depressed people felt significantly less depressed after beginning an
exercise program, compared with those who did not exercise. Regular
workouts, astonishingly enough, were found to be as effective as psychotherapy for depression. Literature reviews consistently indicate that
exercise is associated with reduced stress, higher self-esteem, and
improved body image. The exercise-mood connection is so strong that
the 1996 *U.S. Surgeon General's Report on Physical Activity and Health*
concluded that "physical activity may protect against the development
of depression" and that inactive people have twice the risk of developing depression as active people.

Examine Your Exercising Habits

1. Do you engage in some form of aerobic physical activity (walking, biking, swimming)—that causes you to break a sweat—for thirty minutes or more, at least three times a week?
   a. No   b. Yes

2. Do you engage in some form of muscle-strengthening exercise (weight lifting, muscle-toning exercises) at least twice a week?
   a. No   b. Yes

3. Do you take vacations centered on physical activity (hiking, skiing, camping)?
   a. No   b. Yes

4. Does your body feel physically fit?
   a. No   b. Yes

5. Are you easily winded by everyday activities, such as climbing one or two flights of stairs or carrying groceries?
   a. Yes   b. No

Count your *a* and *b* answers. If you have more *a*'s than *b*'s, you need to work on improving your physical fitness. Follow the three stages of the exercise program in this chapter, and be sure to concentrate your efforts on Stage 1—Learning the Basics— before moving on to Stage 2. If you have more *b*'s than *a*'s, you may be in fairly good physical condition, but perhaps you forget to stretch or are intimidated by working out with weights. In that case, you should still follow all three stages, but you can start with a higher intensity of activity in Stage 1. My plan is designed for everyone (assuming you do not have a serious medical condition), from couch potatoes to professional athletes. And it's been tailored to work in an integrated fashion with the nutrition plan.

Researchers have begun to document the effect that exercise has on the neurochemistry of mood regulation. Steady exercise—everything from Rollerblading to running—activates the sympathetic nervous system, which speeds up your heart rate, breathing, and pulse, increasing blood flow to your muscles and brain, and triggering the release of adrenaline and glucose into your bloodstream. Your brain cells react to this heightened state of activity by releasing endorphins, which are given credit for inducing "the runner's high." Exercise may also boost your mood by influencing the availability and metabolism of serotonin and other neurotransmitters in a way similar to that of antidepressants!

Exercise's effects on your psyche, though, are more than just the sum of your brain chemicals. Exercise may give you a sense of control over your life, or it may distract you from worries. It gives you mastery over a sport and improves your body image. It can provide you with a social support system if you're working out with a partner or group. It also gets you active, which you may view as "doing something" as opposed to "doing nothing." Exercise will help you feel better about yourself because you'll know you're doing something that's good for your body as well as your mind.

Most important, exercise will start you on the road to feeling younger and having a vibrant, active, engaged life.

And you don't need to work out hard and fast to feel good. Research suggests that developing muscular fitness through strength training can make you feel stronger, more powerful, and happier. A study from Brigham Young University in Utah found that sedentary women who participated in a resistance training program for twelve weeks experienced improved body image and self-esteem—even if they didn't lose any weight. The researchers concluded that this is because strength training produces results that can be measured in terms of muscle definition and the amount of weight one can lift.

What all this means is that exercise can help amplify the effects of antidepressants. What's more, it can help you burn off excess pounds that you may have gained as a result of taking antidepressants, can give you more energy, and can improve your sex life. This is why I developed an exercise plan tailored for people who are on antidepressants. This three-stage exercise program can be particularly helpful because it

* boosts energy by improving your immune function, increasing your metabolism, and making everyday tasks seem easier
* enhances sexual function by increasing blood flow to your sex organs
* increases sex drive (if you don't overstrain yourself) by decreasing the production of stress hormones
* fosters weight loss by burning off fat, helping to reduce or maintain appetite, and building up calorie-burning muscles
* helps with weight maintenance by increasing metabolism
* improves circulation, which can bolster the effects of antidepressants

If you're like most of my patients, you probably haven't made exercise a number-one priority in your life. Yet that's exactly what it must be, because your future, and the kind of life you enjoy, depends on it. Many of my patients tell me they're too tired to exercise—often because of the energy drain caused by their antidepressants, stress, and diet. *Whatever your reason for not exercising, you're making a grave mistake, forgoing the very thing that will boost your energy and banish your daily slumps.*

As I was writing this chapter, I received a visit from an old patient named Nick, who illustrates just how well my exercise program works. Nick, a thirty-eight-year-old businessman with a boyish way about him, has been following the Antidepressant Survival Program for the past four years and has found that exercise has given him a new outlook. I asked Nick to compare his life before exercise and after he began working out. "Before I got into shape, my medications [Prozac and Xanax] had flipped the off switch on panic attacks and depression, but they also flipped the switch on my energy and sex drive." He continued with a twinkle in his eye, "Exercise turned me back on."

Nick had been off and on the antidepressants for eight years before I finally convinced him to try my program. While following the nutrition plan, he began strength training and biking fifteen miles to work. After a few weeks he saw a substantial change: "My energy bounced back, my sex life improved, and I noticed that I didn't have the morning mood swings. But even more than that, I found that I just felt better about myself." Nick pronounced those words with his boyish grin and a chuckle that said, in effect, "Hey, I don't understand it, but what the hell, it works!"

Nick decided to move to California and start his own business, something he'd always wanted but never had the confidence to do. His new exercise routine includes surfing at the beach for two hours every morning before work. "Are there days I don't want to exercise? Definitely. But I remember that I always feel great afterwards and that gives me the incentive to get out of bed instead of pushing the snooze button." By his own account, exercise clearly improved Nick's response to the antidepressants and eliminated their sexual side effects. Clearly, the medications could take him only so far: he had to take some steps to get the full life he desired.

BEGIN THE EXERCISE PROGRAM AND NUTRITION PLAN SIMULTANEOUSLY

Exercise is, of course, part of the balanced Fundamentals. It works in concert with the nutrition plan to reduce the side effects you're experiencing from antidepressants and to amplify the effects of the medications. Both alter the workings of your neurotransmitters to improve your moods. Exercise also increases the blood flow to your brain, so your brain cells can get the oxygen and nutrients needed to function at their best. Exercise works together with the nutrition plan to regulate your blood-sugar levels, which helps stabilize your moods and gives you a sustained level of energy.

The exercise program and nutrition plan also go hand in hand in helping you lose excess weight. Eating the proper amount of protein and carbohydrates will provide fuel for your muscle cells while you're strength training and fuel for your heart muscle while you're doing steady exercise. As you gain muscle your metabolism will increase and you'll burn off more calories. Fueling your body with the proper nutrients will also allow you to exert the maximum amount of effort during your workouts, which will boost your weight-loss efforts.

HOW AEROBIC AND WEIGHT TRAINING BALANCE YOUR BODY

I've designed a program that will give you the maximum benefits from exercise by allowing it to work its magic in two distinct ways: increasing your aerobic fitness (which strengthens your heart muscle, improves your circulation, and stabilizes your moods) and building your strength (which adds tone to the rest of your muscles and creates support for your joints and bones). Both work together to improve your physical fitness and mental well-being. Both help you overcome the side effects of antidepressants and get the maximum benefits from the medications. Ultimately, one of the best paths to a fit mind is through a fit body.

Doing a combination of strength training and aerobic exercise will give you a built-in energy advantage. Strength training builds your muscle cells and enables them to make more of the cellular energy factories, called mitochondria. Mitochondria convert sugar to energy. The more of these factories each muscle cell has, the more energy it has at its disposal. Aerobic activity causes your body to sprout new capillaries, tiny blood vessels that bring oxygen to cells. The more oxygen your cells get, the better equipped they are for using fuel, which increases the efficiency of energy production. Beyond these cellular changes, you'll find you have more energy simply because you'll have an easier time performing simple tasks like climbing the stairs or carrying packages in from the supermarket. You may also find that you're feeling more rested, since exercise can help you sleep better by reducing stress and regulating your natural biorhythms. *You shouldn't, however, work out within three hours of bedtime because doing so can disrupt sleep.*

Getting physically fit will also give you a feeling of power, a vital life force that goes hand in hand with energy. Going through depression or a painful medical condition can rob you of a sense of power. You may have been feeling helpless for so long that you've forgotten what it feels like to be in charge of your body and health, to feel powerful. As you increase the amount of weight you lift or bike a little farther, you'll feel stronger and more powerful. You'll even be more motivated to stay on the nutrition plan because you'll know that you're eating to add high-quality fuel to your power source.

You'll also feel more in control of your weight, which may have ballooned as a result of both depression and taking antidepressants. The combination of steady exercise and strength training delivers a one-two punch to your fat cells: Aerobic workouts burn off excess calories, which can mobilize your fat cells to release fat. In addition, your metabolism will remain elevated for several hours after a workout and your appetite will be suppressed temporarily (if you do moderate exercise)—both of which can nudge weight loss further along. Strength training builds up muscle cells, which use more energy than fat cells, so your body needs to burn more calories to keep your muscle cells nourished. These cellular workings are your body's natural way of helping you lose weight.

The typical aerobic workout in Stage 1 of my plan burns 250 to 300 calories. If you continue to eat the same number of calories, you'll burn off a pound (which contains 3,500 calories) over twelve to fifteen workouts. *Remember: The goal is fitness, not weight loss* (although you will lose weight slowly and steadily—and keep it off). If you're doing aerobic workouts four times a week, you'll burn off about a pound a month. What's more, adding muscle mass through strength training can boost your metabolism. You'll not only burn extra calories while you're working out and afterward (this is called the afterburn effect), but adding muscle will help you burn calories faster even at rest.

In getting you to exercise, my goal is to redistribute your body mass, not to put you on a regimented weight-loss plan where you tally the calories you need to burn in order to lose a set number of pounds. *Do not* use the scale as a way to monitor your progress; rather, notice your clothing as it becomes looser around your waist. Over time you'll lose fat until eventually your weight loss tapers off. This means you're taking in and burning off the calories your body needs to sustain its new weight. Exercise then becomes an extremely important tool for preventing a return of depression, as well as weight—a particular challenge for those who take antidepressants. A study of 150 people conducted by Kaiser Permanente in Northern California found that 90 percent of those who maintained their weight loss months after losing weight were exercising at least three times a week for thirty minutes or more; in contrast, only 34 percent of those who regained their weight had been getting regular physical activity.

Exercise will dramatically alter the shape of your body and the way you view your image in the mirror. Your waist will get smaller, your abdomen will become flatter, and your body will look more defined. You will be tightening your belt more and more to keep your skirt or pants snug. As you become physically active, you will begin to notice small things that you can do with ease, such as running up a flight of stairs. You'll enjoy the sense of speed as you run or bike masterfully around a corner. The combination of aerobic and muscle-strengthening exercise will help you turn back the clock and restore a youthful body and mind. In fact, you may find that you look and feel better than you did when you were younger.

Will this newly fit body help improve your sex life? Researchers are beginning to find evidence that this is the case. A 1994 survey of 8,000 women, who said they exercised three to five times a week, found that 40 percent said a light workout made them more easily aroused, 31 percent said exercising increased their frequency of sex, and 27 percent said it enabled them to climax more easily. The vast majority of the respondents said that exercise improved their body images. Exercise can even have immediate benefits: In a recent study researchers showed erotic films to women who had low sexual desire or trouble achieving orgasm. When these women exercised on treadmills just before watching the films, they reported more arousal than when they did not exercise.

Other research has found that exercise can help improve sexual function in men who are having trouble maintaining erections. Exercise can control or reduce numerous factors that impede blood flow to the sex organs. These factors include stress, high blood pressure, high cholesterol, and diabetes. What's more, exercise can boost the sex drive in both men and women by regulating the release of the stress hormone cortisol, which then enables the release of higher levels of sex hormones.

WHAT EXERCISE HAS DONE FOR MY PATIENTS

Michael, a thirty-five-year-old math professor, came to me eight years ago suffering from anxiety and depression. I prescribed Paxil, which helped get his anxiety and depression under control. But Michael told me he now had a new problem: He was tired all the time and frequently fell asleep while grading papers in the evening. He told me he was too tired to think about having sex with his partner, and he was discouraged by his ten-pound weight gain, which occurred after he began taking his antidepressant. I told Michael about the program and advised him he needed to change his nutrition habits and get started on an exercise regimen.

I insisted Michael hire a personal trainer, who created a workout plan that included long-distance running (which Michael used to do in college) interspersed with weight training. After a few weeks of exercising and following the program, Michael told me that he had more energy than he could ever remember having. His sex drive had bounced back as well. "I used to force myself to have sex once or twice a month," he said, "but now I feel the urge to have sex two or three times a week."

Although Michael adhered to his aerobic workouts, he found he had developed a real passion for weight training. He invested in a set of free weights and a weight bench and began to train three or four times a week. Within a few months Michael had lost the ten pounds of fat he had gained and had added pounds of new muscle. Eventually he began to enter weight lifting competitions. He told me that competing made him feel like he was overcoming his childhood sense of smallness and physical failure, and that he had gained a confidence in himself that he never knew he had in him. With his newfound energy he was able to get his own business off the ground (his third attempt), and he now has more business than he can handle. When I told Michael I was writing a book about my program, I asked him what he had gotten out of it. "It showed me that I'm a powerful person," he said. "No challenge is insurmountable."

I had a tougher time convincing another patient to begin exercising. Andrew had developed chronic fatigue syndrome around the time he turned forty, and he was so exhausted he had to quit the firm where he worked as an attorney. His marriage troubles, which had been getting worse over the years, came to a head; his wife decided she wanted a divorce and was granted sole custody of their four children. Andrew sank into a deep depression and came to me for help. I put him on

Prozac, and that helped improve his moods, but he still felt like he could barely lift himself out of bed in the morning. He told me he was certain he had some incurable illness.

I explained to Andrew the concepts of the Antidepressant Survival Program, and he began to balance his protein and carbohydrates more effectively, went through the Medical Prescription portion of the program, and even incorporated the strategies for relaxation and play. He couldn't, however, get himself to exercise more than once or twice a month. He told me he just couldn't seem to get motivated to go biking when it was cold or rainy or to use the set of weights in his basement. I convinced Andrew to join a health club that offered him a variety of workout options. He eventually found he loved taking spinning classes on the bikes and was able to follow a resistance training routine on the Nautilus machines.

After several weeks Andrew began to notice a significant increase in his energy, and within four months he interviewed with a law firm and wound up taking a job there. "I never thought that exercising could be a great way to socialize, but I made some new friends at the health club who didn't immediately see me as a guy down on his luck. Now we go mountain biking together on the weekends when I'm not out camping with my kids." Andrew has learned that exercise needs to come first and must be a routine part of his day. "I know that good nutrition and my supplements are essential, but exercise is what keeps me from slipping back into my chronic fatigue, and I know that I won't be any good to my family or co-workers if I'm not good to myself. I decided that I had to build my life around exercise. I even moved to a different town house to be closer to my health club." Andrew had become the architect of his life.

Andrew is someone I can really relate to. I myself stopped exercising for several years, and I found it virtually impossible to begin again. Ever since my Little League days I had been involved in one sport or another. I played tennis and jogged pretty regularly through college and the first two years of medical school, although I kept up my exercise habits only off and on during the remaining years of med school and residency training.

When I began to practice medicine, I became more diligent about my exercise. I joined a local health club and started to play racquetball.

I took the game pretty seriously, improving my technique and enjoying the vigorous, sweat-filled workouts, until one day I felt a pop and my knee gave way. After surgery to repair my knee, I became somewhat of a couch potato while my body was on the mend. Well after my knee had healed, I couldn't seem to restart my fitness routine. I can't play racquetball anymore, I thought, so what else is there? In keeping with my approach to life, I decided to wait until a new physical interest became clear to me. So I waited, and I waited. Then I waited some more. While waiting I gained a new wardrobe, as well as twenty pounds or more of fat.

Finally, after three years of waiting for the motivation and interest to come to me, I realized that I would never get motivated on my own. I thought about hiring a personal trainer, but I resisted that solution. I thought, This is too Hollywood. Do I really need someone to teach me how to exercise when I can just do it on my own? But I realized a trainer offered me a way around the boredom of weight training—I had forgotten how much I used to enjoy weights in high school. I knew that if I had an appointment to keep, I would actually exercise. I also knew that a trainer could get me started slowly, so I wouldn't overdo it and injure myself in the first few weeks.

I met with the trainer, someone I knew from my racquetball days and felt like I clicked with (which is very important). We met a few times a week for the first few months. (I eventually eased back in frequency as I grew comfortable with my workouts.) The trainer set me up with a routine that involved free weights, weight machines, and biking on an exercise bike. I have to admit that the first few weeks were pretty difficult: The exercise bike was nearly impossible to pedal—all I could think about was the physical fatigue and how much I wanted to quit. I was able to bear my aerobic workouts only by watching TV, reading books, or listening to music.

After six weeks, though, I found that the workouts were much easier and that I was able to push myself harder and faster to feel that "exercise high." I still often needed diversions to get me through my workouts, but more and more frequently I was able to focus on my pedaling and actually began to practice a form of moving meditation.

Slowly, I expanded the activities I was involved in. After one year I started taking hikes with my wife, kids, and dog on the weekends and mountain biking with a friend. Now, five years later, I still meet with my trainer for evaluation sessions, or for a new weight training routine, every one to three months, as I feel the need. I'm also continuing to expand my exercise horizons: I've taken a sculling class taught by the coach of the local university crew team.

Unless there's a medical reason not to, I insist that all my patients exercise. After I give my patients my spiel about the importance of exercise, many of them turn to me and say, "Doc, I'm really going to try." I tell them, "That's not good enough. I want to know when you're going to buy a new pair of sneakers and what day you're planning to start your first workout. I want to know what you will do, for how long, and what your goal is for the next time we meet. Then I want you to promise me that you'll stick with those commitments."

The truth is that "trying" is just not going to cut it. "I'll try to get there on time" means you may find an excuse to be twenty minutes late. Saying to yourself that you'll try to exercise means that you are retaining the option of finding a "good" reason not to. To "try" is to fail. If I may paraphrase the character Yoda from the movie *The Empire Strikes Back:* "There is no try. There is only Do or Not Do."

GETTING INTO THE EXERCISE MIND-SET

In this life, each of us is the author of our personal journey. We are the designers of our own lives, giving them direction, structure, and form, in the same way that an artist creates a work of art or an architect designs a building. *You* are the architect of your life. Once you commit yourself to a goal, you will achieve it. Note, however, that committing to a goal is very different from wishing or wanting to achieve a goal. "I wish I was exercising" or "I want to exercise" is very different from "I will exercise." "I wish I could stop eating chocolate" or "I want to stop eating chocolate" is very different from "I will stop eating chocolate." Say these statements out loud or silently, now, and notice the difference in how you feel. Do this before you continue to read.

Mental Exercise

1. Sit in a comfortable chair, and relax.
2. Take three deep breaths, and then close your eyes.

3. Think to yourself "I *wish* I _____."
   (Fill in the blank with what you wish for, such as "I wish I could exercise.")
4. Repeat the statement to yourself and notice how you feel.
5. Open your eyes.
6. Now, take three more deep breaths, close your eyes, and think "I *am* _____."
   (e.g., going to exercise)
7. Notice the difference in how you feel now. That is the power of thought.

If you suffered from depression or a chronic illness, you've probably felt helpless for so long that it's hard to acknowledge that you now have more control over your life. Maybe you've never experienced the right balance of nutrition, exercise, and happiness. Maybe you've never made yourself a number-one priority. This may sound like a cliché, but I believe it is very true. You must take care of yourself first—which means learning and making the Fundamentals a routine part of your life, like sleeping.

The good news is you've already begun to put yourself first. You've taken the step to get treatment for your medical condition, which is why you're on antidepressants. These medications will help you overcome the inertia that set in from your previous medical condition. You've also taken the initiative to read this book. You may have put yourself through the Jump Start, which gave you a taste for the full program.

So you see, you've already shifted yourself into gear. Now it's time to get yourself moving. You've begun to shed your helpless self and are ready to wrap yourself in your new willful, powerful persona.

Realizing that exercise may be either entirely new to you or a faded memory from the past, I've designed a program to ease you into exercise in three stages. With each stage you will master a new set of skills, and by the end of the program you'll be fit enough to take on any activity you choose. You may think that you're "not the athletic type" or that exercise "just isn't fun." (These were two reasons women cited for not exercising in a recent poll conducted by the Gallup organization and *Health* magazine.) This plan will prove to you that you can overcome these barriers, that you can find the athlete hidden within you, and that you will have fun once you learn the basics. The key is to choose some activity that's easy enough to master and that's potentially enjoyable. Remember, all the elements of the Fundamentals are part of a long-term plan designed to give you pleasure. Once you start your exercise program, remember to keep your goals flexible. If you feel tired one day, back off on the exercise intensity. If you are scheduled to work out in the gym but it's a beautiful day, take a brisk walk instead. You cannot and should not be a robot or a slave to anything or anyone—including exercise. The point is to develop an active lifestyle, one that stimulates your body and mind. Just like in everything else in life, variety, novelty, and spontaneity are welcome companions. So if you come across a scenic view while you're riding your bike or jogging outdoors, take the time to stop and enjoy it.

Note: Check with your doctor before beginning this exercise program. You may need to show your doctor the plan to have it modified to fit your particular health needs.

STAGE 1:
LEARNING THE BASICS

You've gotten a feel for exercise on the Jump Start. You got yourself moving, and you may already have experienced exercise's energizing and mood-boosting effects. Now it's time to incorporate exercise into your life and improve your physical fitness. Stage 1 is designed to introduce you to aerobic activity and strength training. You should work up your activity slowly during this stage, which lasts about six weeks. If you've already been exercising, begin at your current time and intensity level and gradually increase. If you've always been a committed couch potato, increase the time and intensity of your workouts gradually, so you feel like you're pushing yourself but not overdoing it.

The goal of Stage 1 is to master one aerobic activity and get comfortable with strength training. (If you try to take on too many activities at once, you may get frustrated or increase the likelihood of injuries.) Stage 2, which also lasts approximately six weeks, will introduce you to cross training and allow you to vary your aerobic activities.

Stage 3 is a maintenance plan, to keep you from slipping off the fitness track over the long term.

You should begin to feel more energy and an improvement in your moods almost immediately. And you will be amazed at how quickly your stamina increases. One patient told me she could barely make it around the block the first day. After only four weeks she was walking around the block four times and now was looking for a bigger block. I remember when I was in medical school studying ten hours a day for my board exams. I needed a way to release the tension and get some physical activity, so I started jogging. I could barely run the distance between telephone poles, so I would run one "pole" and walk one "pole." I remember being surprised how soon I was able to run two poles, then three, then the entire distance.

Begin the exercise program at the same time you begin the nutrition plan. This will enable you to experience the full mood-boosting and energizing benefits that occur when you properly fuel your body with the right foods and activities.

Aerobic Activity

Choose *one* aerobic activity from this list:
Brisk walking or hiking (outside or on the treadmill)
Jogging (outside or on the treadmill)
Swimming
Water aerobics
Outdoor biking or stationary biking
Climbing stairs (in your house, office, or on a stair climber), or climbing hills
Jumping rope
Rowing machine, or rowing
Ski machine, or cross-country skiing
Fast dancing to music (at home or in a dance class)
Aerobics class at the gym or home video (see Appendix One for suggestions)

Note: I didn't include recreational activities (horseback riding, baseball, basketball, and so on) because many of them do not keep your heart rate elevated consistently, so they're not likely to give you the mood-boosting effects of exercise. If you are already engaged in an aerobic activity that's not on this list, feel free to use that activity for your aerobic choice.

Strength Training

The goal is to build strength and tone muscles (though not bulk) at this point in the program. You need to aim for more repetitions (twelve to fifteen) at a lighter weight to increase your overall muscle tone. (Doing fewer repetitions at a higher weight tends to increase bulk, which should not be attempted until Stage 2. Bulking up is more likely to result in injury—especially if you haven't done some basic conditioning and worked on your flexibility.) Most important, remember that using good form is a higher priority than the amount of weight lifted or the number of repetitions performed. See Appendix One for recommended resistance training books.

Whenever doing muscle-strengthening exercises, you should use enough resistance that your muscles feel fatigued and even burning (during the final repetitions of each set) but not in pain afterward. You can use free weights, weight machines (such as Nautilus or Cybex), or exercise bands, depending on what appeals to you. I strongly recommend starting Stages 1 and 2 of the program with weight machines to reduce your chance of injury and help you develop proper form. You'll see that your strength will improve fairly quickly. Research suggests that the average adult can expect a 25 percent improvement in strength within the first two months of starting a resistance training program.

As your strength improves, you'll want to increase the number of sets. I want you to work up to three sets of fifteen repetitions, comfortably done with very good form (smooth and slow on both contraction and release) before increasing your poundage.

If you don't have access to a gym, dumbbells are a reasonable way to get started. A good starter set of dumbbells includes pairs of two, three, five, eight, ten, twelve, fifteen, and twenty pounds. You also need a comfortable weight bench for moves that require lying down, kneeling, or leaning back.

How do you get started? Find a trainer to teach you the basics. If this is not possible, purchase a how-to book or video for diagrammed moves that work all your major muscle groups. One good book is *Weight Training for Dummies* (IDG Books, 1997) by Liz Neporent and Suzanne Schlosberg. For videos try anything by Gilad, Kathy Smith, or Gin Miller that's geared to beginners.

What will it cost? Although weight sets can run into the hundreds of dollars, you can buy a standard set of dumbbells for as little as fifty to one hundred dollars (you can even check the local classifieds for good deals). A standard weight bench complete with a barbell and weights can be purchased for a hundred dollars in discount sports stores.

FLEXIBILITY

Stretching is often the forgotten fitness factor, but it is important for a fit and balanced body. When you age you naturally lose flexibility as muscle fibers and tendons shorten. As a result, your body doesn't move as freely, which can make you uncomfortable and more prone to injuries, particularly in your lower back. The good news is you can prevent some of aging's muscle-restricting effects through stretching. It's best to target the major tight spots: the upper and lower back and shoulders, the arms (biceps and triceps), the chest, and the legs (quadriceps, hamstrings, calves, and hips).

Before stretching spend five to ten minutes walking, jogging, or riding a stationary bike at a gentle pace. This will get the blood flowing and the heart pumping, and warm up your muscles, making it safer to stretch them. (Stretching a cold muscle increases the chances of tearing muscle fibers.) When performing a stretch, stretch to the point where you feel mild tension, not pain, in your muscles. Hold the stretch for thirty seconds. (Don't bounce to stretch a muscle. Bouncing can cause injury by rapidly placing too much tension on the muscle.) Stretch just before and after working each muscle group.

A SIX-WEEK WORKOUT PLAN

In just six weeks the three-times-a-week aerobic exercise regimen (the activity you chose from the earlier list) and the twice-a-week strength training regimen will help you learn the exercise fundamentals. You'll notice that I've given you two rest days a week. You can take your rest days on any day that you choose. Just make sure you don't have two

Getting Set to Exercise:
A Checklist

Now that you've got a game plan for what you're going to do, I want you to figure out how you're going to do it. Fill in this exercise planner.

1. Aerobic exercise you plan to do:

   _____

2. Type of weights you plan to use:

   _____

3. Exercise gear you plan to buy (sneakers, weights, pulse monitor, a notepad to record your workouts, and so on):

   _____

   _____

   _____

   _____

4. Days and times you plan to exercise:

Sunday _____

Monday _____

Tuesday _____

Wednesday _____

Thursday _____

Friday _____

Saturday _____

5. Your Stage 1 goals:

Aerobic _____

Resistance _____

6. Situations in which you are likely to miss exercise, and
   coping strategy:

   _____

   _____

   _____

   _____

   _____

   _____

7. People who will be likely to support your exercise:

   _____

   _____

8. People who will be likely to undermine your exercise, and
   how you plan to cope with them:

   _____

   _____

	Weeks 1 and 2	Weeks 3 and 4	Weeks 5 and 6
Sunday	Aerobic activity 20–25 minutes	Aerobic activity 30–35 minutes	Aerobic activity 40–45 minutes
Monday	Strength train, 1 set 12–15 repetitions	Strength train, 1–2 sets 12–15 reps	Strength train, 2–3 sets 12–15 reps
Tuesday	Rest	Rest	Rest
Wednesday	Aerobic activity 20–25 minutes	Aerobic activity 30–35 minutes	Aerobic activity 40–45 minutes
Thursday	Strength train, 1 set, 12–15 reps	Strength train, 2 sets 12–15 reps	Strength train, 3 sets 12–15 reps
Friday	Rest	Rest	Rest
Saturday	Aerobic activity 20–25 minutes	Aerobic activity 30–35 minutes	Aerobic activity 40–45 minutes

back-to-back days of resistance training for the same muscle group. (Muscles need a day off to repair themselves from the minuscule tears that occur when you build them up.)

Note: To reduce your risk of injury and increase your flexibility, begin your workouts with a five- to ten-minute warm-up and end with a five- to ten-minute cool-down. Always do your stretches before and after exercising each muscle group.

Keep a daily exercise diary or notebook. Write down what exercise you did and for how long. Record the amount of weight you lifted and the number of repetitions and sets. Rate your workouts on a scale of 1 to 5, with 1 being the least intense and 5 being the most intense. Are you scoring mostly 1's and 2's? If so, you need to increase the length or the intensity of your workouts. If you're scoring mostly 5's, you need to cut back.

Important hint: You may not be having much fun—you may even dread your workouts—as you begin to integrate exercise into your life. If this is so, chances are you are the type of person who likes familiarity and avoids what you perceive to be a potentially harmful or painful situation. Your enjoyment of exercise will increase as you master your workouts and they become a routine part of your life.

Try smiling while you work out. You'll be surprised by the mood-boosting effects. And think positive. Say to yourself, "This is good. I will do it." Some people set imaginary incentives: "If I do the next set, I'm going to win a million dollars."

An amazing study found that elderly people in nursing homes who worked out with weights were able to increase their muscle mass at the same rate as twenty-five-year-olds who were put on the same weight training regimen. Nature is ready to work for you—no matter what your age!

Do not focus on weight loss! Weight loss will come gradually and naturally. Let the fit of your clothes, your endurance, and your resting pulse serve as your guides.

Remember to drink plenty of water, and if you have low blood pressure, eat plenty of salt! Once you begin exercising you will be losing a lot of water during and shortly after your workouts. You'll probably feel thirsty (which means you're already a little dehydrated). You need to keep yourself well hydrated by drinking about eight glasses of water daily—preferably early in the day, so you are hydrated before you exercise and are not spending your nights in the bathroom. Keeping your water intake up will help you avoid light-headedness, dizziness, fatigue, and difficulty recovering from exercise sessions.

Eat a light snack about an hour before you exercise to give your body energy. Make sure it contains both protein and carbohydrates. A good snack: carrot and celery sticks with cottage cheese, or, if you are on the run, try a Balance bar (a nutrition bar available in health-food stores). After you exercise replenish your body stores by eating another protein-carbohydrate snack. Listen to your body—if you notice you are craving salty foods, increase the salt in your diet (unless your doctor advises against it because of other health considerations).

STAGE 2: CROSS TRAINING

Once you've mastered an aerobic activity, you'll begin to enjoy the benefits of a toned body. Now, you're ready to take on two new aerobic activities, which will enable you to cross train. Cross training varies your workouts to make them less monotonous and enables you to work different muscle groups. If you continue your same exercise routine without increasing the intensity or type of activity, your muscles will deal with the exercise stress more efficiently and you won't get as much of a workout. To keep improving your fitness, you need to take on some new challenges.

In this stage of the program, you will achieve mastery over three different aerobic activities and expand your horizons. This is a time to do something that you may have never done on a regular basis. You'll be giving yourself a chance to see which activities you enjoy the most.

You will also increase the weight in your strength training regimen. Go up one dumbbell size, go down a notch on your Nautilus machine, or add five-pound weights to your barbells. Remember, do more repetitions (twelve to fifteen) and use less weight if you want to tone up without bulking up. If you want to increase muscle bulk, do three sets of strength training exercises consisting of eight to ten repetitions for each major muscle group in the legs, arms, back, chest, and abdomen two or three times per week.

PLAN FOR CROSS TRAINING

Let's say you were walking during Stage 1. Now you've decided to bike and take some aerobics classes. Here's what your plan would look like.

	Weeks 1 and 2	Weeks 3 and 4	Weeks 5 and 6
Sunday	Walk 50 minutes	Walk 55 minutes	Walk 1 hour
Monday	Strength train, 3 sets 8–12 reps or 12–15 reps	Strength train, 3 sets 8–12 reps or 12–15 reps	Strength train, 3 sets 8–12 reps or 12–15 reps
Tuesday	Rest	Rest	Rest
Wednesday	Bike 25–35 minutes	Bike 40–50 minutes	Bike 55–60 minutes
Thursday	Strength train, 1 set 8–12 reps or 12–15 reps	Strength train, 1–2 sets 8–12 reps or 12–15 reps	Strength train, 2–3 sets 8–12 reps or 12–15 reps
Friday	Rest	Rest	Rest
Saturday	Aerobics class (beginners)	Aerobics class (intermediate)	Aerobics class (advanced)

This phase of the program can be as short as six weeks or as long as twenty-four. *Find your own pace. You will know you have completed this phase when you are comfortable in the activities you're doing.* Your goal is one hour of each aerobic activity each week.

Note: You can split your workouts into two or three different activities, say, alternating five minutes on the stationary bike with five minutes on the treadmill. Or you can just do a different activity each time you work out.

STAGE 3:
MAINTENANCE

After you finish Stage 2, you'll be able to pat yourself on the back for a job well done. You'll feel a *major* difference in your body and mood, and people around you will be commenting on how great you look. You'll have gotten yourself into good physical condition, but you'll still face your greatest challenge: *maintaining your exercise habits.* The fact is that half of all people who start a new exercise program quit within six months.

Stop here and think. *Decide* whether you will be an exercise quitter or an exercise lifer. Affirm your commitment by saying to yourself, "I now commit to some form of exercise for life." On one occasion I found myself wondering how I would go about doing isometric exercises if, in my old age, I were in a wheelchair. (I'm an exercise lifer.)

Like many neophyte fitness buffs, you may have been really gung ho during Stages 1 and 2 of my exercise program. Unfortunately, it's all too easy to lose your momentum: You take a vacation, are stressed at home or work, or are laid up for a week with the flu or a pulled muscle. You've broken your fitness routine, and your old sedentary habits reemerge. You just can't seem to bring yourself to start your workouts back up again.

Injury is a common reason people stop exercising. As I related in my own experience with exercise, injury can set you on the exercise sidelines for months or years. The key is to look for an alternative activity that won't aggravate your injury. (You should, of course, have your injury evaluated by your doctor and get recommendations for substitute activities that won't worsen the injury.) Fortunately, most injuries won't waylay you from all activities. For instance, if your knees are sore from jogging, take up a low-impact activity like swimming, biking, or brisk walking. If you've strained your lower back, try a stationary recumbent bike or swimming until it heals.

Even if you don't suffer an injury or other acute setback, you may simply find that you begin skipping a workout or two a week when other demands on your time become "urgent," or you have a cold. Pretty soon you're exercising only a few times a month, and then you drop exercise from your life altogether. Stage 3 is about finding a way to overcome the ultimate exercise obstacle: *boredom.* It's about building in alternatives to your ho-hum exercise routine.

You may find that you've walked too many miles, swum too many laps, or climbed too many steps on the StairMaster. *It's time to start varying your workout routine!* During Stages 1 and 2 you mastered three different aerobic activities. In Stage 3 I'd like you to get a taste for the vast world of "fitness fun." Fitness fun is anything that gets you active while allowing you to have an adventurous and enjoyable experience. You may even find that one of the new activities you try can be incorporated into your regular fitness routine. This is the time to vary your experiences and shake up your exercise routine. You'll be having fun while working different muscles and continuing to improve your fitness.

In Stage 3

* Continue to follow the exercise plan from Stage 2.
* Once a month add in a novel fitness fun activity (from the following list). You can use it to replace your usual aerobic workout or do it on a rest day. *Look for opportunities to do anything new with someone who can teach and guide you.*
* Consider marathons, group activities, or lessons to get you started.
* Every six weeks, meet with a "fitness support" person to reevaluate your fitness goals. This can be a trainer, your therapist, or a friend or loved one (preferably someone whose exercise you can monitor as well).
* Go over your resistance training routine. Can you increase to the next size in dumbbells or go up to a higher weight on the Nautilus machines? This is a good time to incorporate one of the fitness fun activities you have tried and liked into your regular exercise program.

Fitness Fun Activities

These are just a few suggestions.

Outdoor (Spring, Summer, Fall)

Nature walking
Hiking
Rollerblading

Mountain biking
Baseball or softball
Tennis
Touch football or Frisbee
Beach volleyball
Surfing
Sailing
Canoeing
Kayaking
Sculling
White-water rafting
Rock climbing
Outdoor exercise club (hiking, biking, runners' clubs)
Horseback riding
Scuba diving or snorkeling

Outdoor (Winter)

Ice skating
Snowshoeing
Downhill or cross-country skiing
Ice hockey
Tubing
Snowboarding
Building a snowman or an igloo

Indoor

Basketball
Tennis
Martial arts class (karate, tae kwon do, judo)
Tai chi or yoga
Slow body movement class
Modern dance class
Rock-climbing wall
Boxing or kick boxing
Squash
Racketball
Gymnastics

Tips for Maximizing Your Chances of Exercise Success

Give up the guilt. We are all bound to miss a week or two of exercise when we get sick or go on vacation. Feeling guilty will only damage your self-esteem. As a motivational tool, think back to how good you felt when you were exercising. Remember, you can feel this way again once you get moving. Even better, ask a friend or trainer to remind you to restart your program ahead of time.

Use a short workout to keep you on track. If you don't have time for your standard workout one day, do a few push-ups in your office, or keep a jump rope in your desk drawer that you can use for an intensive "on the fly" workout when time is limited. Do a few minutes of jumping jacks or some abdominal crunches in front of the television.

Use exercise cues. Put Post-it notes on your refrigerator, phones, car windshield, and desk at work with little reminders to exercise like "Go to the gym!" or "Take the stairs—not the elevator!" Put your gym bag on the driver's seat of your car so you can't ignore it at the end of the day. Hang your exercise chart or diary next to your mirror. Be creative with these cues, and plant them where and when you need the impetus most.

Know your weaknesses. Identify high-risk times when you are likely to skip your usual exercise routine and create strategies to squeeze in exercise whenever you can. As I was writing this book, I knew I would have less time to exercise at a health club near my office. I decided to eliminate lunch meetings so I could have more time to exercise.

Associate with people who have an active lifestyle. Social support is a powerful ingredient in making exercise a part of your everyday life. Be aware that some well-meaning but envious people may attempt to undermine your efforts by telling you that exercise is a waste of time or predicting your failure by saying, "Oh, I once worked out all the time. Trust me, it won't last."

Date	Activity	Duration	Pulse*
Sunday, 12/01/99	Running	Ran 10 minutes, walked 20 minutes	115–125
Tuesday, 12/03/99	Running	Ran 12 minutes, walked 18 minutes	113–126
Thursday, 12/05/99	Running	Ran 13 minutes, walked 17 minutes	115–124

*See Monitoring Your Pulse, below.

Sample Resistance Training Chart

Date	Exercise	Weight	Repetitions	Sets
Monday, 12/02/99	Bicep Curl	25 lb.	15	2
	Tricep Extension	30 lb.	15	2

Get into an exercise mind-set. Going on a cruise or to a hotel on business? Make sure it has a health club—as most do. Want to enjoy the fall foliage? Take a fast walk through the woods instead of a drive.

Keep an exercise diary. A diary or notebook will let you see the progress you are making. As simple as it sounds, *this provides a tremendous incentive to keep exercising.* See the sample above.

Monitoring Your Pulse

Since taking your pulse is often difficult while moving, I strongly recommend you get a pulse monitor from a sports and fitness store or your gym. There are major advantages to using a good pulse monitor. On days when you're energetic, you will not overshoot your target heart rate. On days when you're sluggish, think you're barely making it, and may want to quit, you will be surprised to find that it doesn't take as much effort as you thought to get to your target heart rate and accomplish your goal. This will give you energy, and motivation. It will also teach you about your body.

I'd like you to be working out at 70 percent of your maximum aerobic capacity. This gives you a moderate workout with the best conditioning effects without leading to excess fatigue. At this heart rate you should be breathing heavily but steadily (you shouldn't be gasping for air) and find it somewhat difficult to carry on a conversation. Over time you may find that there is a certain level of intense exercise that absolutely controls your appetite for two or three days at a time.

1. *Calculate your desired pulse.* Subtract your age from 220 and multiply that number by 70 percent. For example, if you are forty years old, $220 - 40 = 180 \times 70\% = 126$ beats per minute. This is your desired pulse rate, within a plus-or-minus-5 range of 121–131.

2. *Take your pulse (if you do not have a pulse monitor).* Find the pulse on your wrist by holding your hand palm side up. Press your index and middle fingers on the spot on the outer third of your wrist, directly below your thumb (about 1 inch down from where your hand meets your wrist). Count the number of beats for 10 seconds. Multiply that number by 6 to get your pulse.

Note: Do not take your pulse at your neck. By doing so you might activate a reflex that can cause you to become light-headed and even faint.

Getting Exercise in Small Doses

On some days you just may not be able to squeeze a half-hour block of time out of your day to exercise. What should you do if you can't fit in a workout? Get your exercise in ten-minute bursts of activity. Recent studies have shown that small amounts of exercise several times a day improve fitness as much as a single daily workout of the same total time. A 1998 study found that exercising in several short rounds over the course of the day helps lower blood fats—which are associated with heart disease and decreased sexual function—as much as one long round. Other research suggests that short bursts of moderate activities can reduce the risk of heart disease, Type 2 diabetes, and some cancers. So if you can't schedule in thirty minutes on the treadmill, try these time savers:

* Take a ten-minute walk during lunch or, even better, climb stairs in the office building for ten minutes.
* Jump rope in a private area for ten minutes. This is a great idea because it is intensive and time limited, and the equipment can be stored anywhere.
* Take your laundry up and down the stairs, one load at a time. (Or find any other excuse to keep going up and down the stairs.)
* While running errands, park several blocks from your destination and walk very briskly the rest of the way.
* Do a quick yard tidy: Pick up any branches; pull a few weeds; trim a few hedges; gather up your children's toys—all in ten minutes.
* Do a scrub down: Clean some old stains off your carpets, your floors, or your bathtub by applying a little elbow grease.

Exercise Danger Signs

When you start exercising, some muscle soreness is almost inevitable as you put your body through moves that it has not encountered in a long time. But you shouldn't be gritting your teeth in pain or feeling the pain intensify as you continue to exercise or after you end your workout. The following are signs that you may have an injury or medical condition that needs to be checked out by a doctor:

Chest pain: Stop exercising immediately. You should have your heart evaluated to rule out heart disease.

Pain that feels knifelike or is focused on one spot: Stop exercising immediately. You may have a tear in a tendon or ligament, caused by poor form, excess weight, or other factors. Have the injury evaluated by your doctor.

Difficulty breathing: If you find yourself gasping for breath with minimal exertion, you may have asthma, lung disease, liver, kidney, or heart disease. Any of these conditions requires immediate evaluation by your doctor.

The Benefits of the Buddy System

Working out with a buddy makes it far more likely that you'll stick with your exercise program, according to studies at the University of Georgia and Stanford University School of Medicine. This is especially true if you're still feeling depressed or have suffered from depression in the past. I highly recommend personal trainers because they can set you up with an individualized fitness plan that's best suited to your preferences and fitness level. They can also work around your schedule and monitor your progress.

Most personal trainers work at health clubs (a major benefit to joining a health club). Still, many trainers are self-employed and are willing to come to your home. You'll pay about forty dollars an hour, according to a survey conducted by IDEA. *Ask for a trainer who is certified by the American College of Sports Medicine or the National Strength and Conditioning Association.*

If you can't afford a personal trainer, find a friend to work out with. Set a schedule that you can both commit to and be each other's trainers. You'll see that you're more motivated to stick to your workouts if you know you'll be letting someone down by canceling, and talking helps the time pass.

SUMMING UP

As you become physically fit, keep in mind that the main point of exercise is to make you feel good. Feeling good involves being healthy and looking your best. It also involves having fun. Exercise should be enjoyable—at least to some degree. I'll be the first to admit that it involves hard work. You'll grunt, sweat, and do a lot of heavy lifting. But I don't want you to feel miserable during your workouts. That's not the point. If you're agonizing through your activities, even after you have mastered them, you need to find a new form of exercise that you can get some enjoyment out of, or find a diversion while you exercise (for instance, books on tape, reading material you would not normally be able to get to).

Remember that all aspects of the Fundamentals are designed to gradually and steadily increase your enjoyment of life. Exercise should be something that you look forward to because you know how good it makes you feel in the rest of your life. If you're having fun while you're working out, so much the better! That's one of the main points of the next chapter: incorporating fun and play into your life.

Over the course of your lifetime, you'll probably be trying different types of exercise. *Be open to change,* and be flexible and creative in your activity choices. Once you've mastered the challenge of keeping exercise in your life, any new form you take on will be a piece of cake.

CHAPTER SIX

Spiritual
Renewal

Relaxation, Play, and Spirituality

* * *

*There is only one purpose for all of life, and
that is for you and all that lives to experience
fullest glory. Everything else you say, think, or
do is attendant to that function. There is
nothing else for your soul to do, and nothing
else your soul wants to do.*

NEALE DONALD WALSCH,
Conversations with God

IF YOU'RE LIKE MOST PEOPLE, you probably lead a high-stress life
in a hectic world, and experiencing pleasure has been relegated to the
bottom of your daily to-do list—behind picking up your dry cleaning,
filing your taxes, and keeping some food in your refrigerator. Your previous depression or physical illness may have robbed you of joy and
contentment.

The preceding chapters provide nourishment for your body and
mind through good nutrition and exercise. The third leg of the
Fundamentals is nourishment for your spirit—equally important to
your fundamental health and well-being, to enjoying a life in balance.

When we talk about the side effects of antidepressants, we usually
think in terms of the physical impacts on sexuality, energy, or weight.
But your spirit is often the victim of collateral damage. Depression is an
isolating and debilitating state during which hope, motivation, and

Assess Your Stress Level

1. When you're stressed, do you try to reduce the stress through a form of relaxation (prayer, meditation, hobbies, pleasurable experience)?
   a. Yes   b. No

2. Are certain components of your life (family, professional, financial, health, relationship, leisure) "under stress" on a routine basis?
   a. No   b. Yes

3. Do you take part in some spiritual activity (for example, prayer, meditation) on a regular basis?
   a. Yes   b. No

4. Would you say that having fun is a high priority in your life?
   a. Yes   b. No

5. Do you view your life's mishaps with humor (rather than sadness or anger)?
   a. Yes   b. No

6. Do you frequently set up your days so that you have something to look forward to?
   a. Yes   b. No

7. Do you have a strong support network of family or friends you can turn to when you're stressed?
   a. Yes   b. No

8. Do you frequently feel isolated or lonely?
   a. No   b. Yes

belief in yourself are vanquished. And while antidepressants help pull you out of the depths of despair, they aren't magic bullets. You need to systematically rebuild and renew your spirit. Take the quiz on the following page. Do you have more *b* than *a* answers? If you're too stressed out to experience pleasure, if you've forgotten how to play and laugh, if you've lost your connection to the people and activities that give you a daily boost, then all the good nutrition and exercise in the world won't bring joy back into your life.

We all have a spiritual life, though yours may have become submerged during your bouts of depression, and subsequently by the side effects of antidepressants. Your spiritual identity may be tied to a formal religion, or it may be secular. But each of us has a best, essential self, which we intuitively recognize as the force within us—or outside us—that animates and gives expression to our lives. Reawakening your dormant spirit—reigniting your divine spark, if you will—is vital to recovering a complete and pleasurable life.

Let me try to be more specific about the goals of the spiritual renewal phase of my program. There are three primary objectives: equilibrium, connection, and pleasure.

Equilibrium is the ability to absorb the shocks of daily life. When you hit a pothole along the way—as we all do, whether at work, with friends, or in the family—you want to roll with the impact and keep on trucking. You'll know you hit something, but you won't go careening off the road. One of the hallmarks of depression is the sense of losing control over your life—your body, your emotions, and your personal direction. While total control is a counterproductive goal, it's important to feel that you're in the driver's seat, not a helpless passenger in your life while it spins out of control in reaction to every crisis.

Connection—to other people, to the community we inhabit, or even to our best inner selves—is vital to our day-to-day happiness. When you were suffering from depression or some other painful medical problem, you probably felt like the Berlin Wall was separating you from your loved ones. (You may even have wanted it there.) You were alone on one side of the wall, while your family and friends stood helplessly by on the other side. You may have felt totally disconnected from the world going on around you as you turned inward to focus on your own problems. You worried about your future and ruminated on regrets about the past. Your thoughts came to be centered on your inhibitions, your limitations, your impending doom—all bricks in the wall that was keeping everyone else out. Antidepressants created a door in that wall. You can now see a way out, a way to reconnect with the greatest joys in your life. *But antidepressants won't take you through the door. You have to walk through it on your own.*

Pleasure—the ability to experience happiness—is what we all want in life. Yet one of the core aspects of depression is most concisely defined as an inability to experience pleasure (anhedonia). Antidepressants can eliminate a lot of barriers to pleasure, but the pleasure pathways in your brain may well have become overgrown and submerged from disuse. I'm not just speaking metaphorically here. It's a well-known medical fact that depression inhibits the ability to experience pleasure. Researchers have been studying this problem for years, and they have been able to map out the exact neurological pathways involved in the experience of pleasure—neural networks that deliver pleasurable neurotransmitters, such as dopamine, in response to pleasurable stimuli. In the depressed state these pleasure pathways become relatively inactive, and sensitivity to all types of pain—both emotional and physical—is increased. Antidepressants can help restore the chemical balance in these pathways, but in order to have ready access to the experience— rather than merely the idea—of pleasure, you need to reactivate these pathways the same way you need to rebuild muscles that have atrophied from a lack of exercise. In this chapter I'll explain how.

But first I'd like to clarify what I mean by *spirituality* in the context of my program. I'm not talking about the kind of mystical transcendence you may have experienced in manic, or even depressed, moments. I'm talking about the small daily epiphanies that give life meaning—the simple moments of connection and joy that come upon us unawares, perhaps when we're kneeling in a backyard garden, feeling the cool earth between our fingers, or merely watching someone we love getting dressed in the morning or sleep at night.

A favorite film moment of mine comes at the end of *Stardust Memories,* when the Woody Allen character (the quintessential anhedonist) is trying to define the meaning of life. He sums it up in the memory of a fleeting moment of sublime happiness: It was a Sunday morning when he was sitting in his apartment, eating yogurt, and watching his girlfriend read the Sunday newspaper. A cool spring breeze wafts through the window, and a Louis Armstrong record he loves is playing in the background. His girlfriend looks up at him, smiles, and returns to her reading. In that moment everything comes together—the music, the breeze, the sunlight, the connection to the woman he loves—and he's happy. For a moment he is living in *now,* not obsessed with the past or the future.

Try this simple exercise in experiencing the *now:* Stop reading at the end of this paragraph and become aware of the sensory ocean surrounding you. Are you in sunlight or lamplight, or some combination? What are the dominant colors of your immediate environment? What can you smell and hear? What messages is your body sending you, either pleasant or unpleasant? Without any conscious thinking, what emotions are you feeling, right now? As religious adepts of every persuasion have reported, there is tremendous freedom in the *now.* You can taste this freedom any time you take the trouble to stop and listen and look and feel. And every time you do this exercise, the experience will be different.

Not exactly a religious experience—no flashes of light or thunderclaps. But in many respects small moments like these are the closest we get to transcendence, to escaping the prison of the past and experiencing the happiness of sensation, emotion, and connection. They're what make life worth living. You don't have to be an artistic genius or a mystic to have access to these moments. But you do need to clear away the clutter of stress and self-centered preoccupation for long enough to let pleasure into your consciousness. If you can relax and enjoy yourself, your spirit will emerge, as if from a deep sleep.

There are three areas of spiritual renewal this chapter focuses on: stress reduction (or relaxation), play (purposeless pleasure), and spirituality (joyous connection). While relaxation, play, and spirituality are all closely related in that they have rejuvenating effects on the spirit, they are also distinct activities. Here's my prescription for spiritual renewal:

1. Spend fifteen minutes a day reducing stress.
2. Actively pursue a playful activity on a daily basis.

3. Incorporate a spiritually renewing pleasure into your daily or weekly routine (such as the *now* exercise performed in your favorite garden, or even a quiet, reflective moment in your favorite room of the house, before the kids wake up in the morning).

THE VALUE OF RELAXATION

Stress and tension are the enemies of relaxation. We all carry around more tension than we realize, and as we become accustomed to it, we notice it less. We carry it in our muscles, in our minds, in our guts, and in our relationships. When we are tense for long periods of time, we feel irritable, withdrawn, and tired. We lose enthusiasm for life. The optimal solution is to reduce the sources of stress in our lives, but on a practical level that's not always possible. We need to make a living, support and care for a family. Adult life tends to be stressful. A more pragmatic approach to stress reduction is to learn to "relax on demand."

What is relaxation? Relaxation is the art of letting go. It is the act of releasing tension from your muscles and sweeping away troubling thoughts from your mind. Both the mind and the body need to be free from stress in order to achieve a state of relaxation. Relaxation is more than just taking a bubble bath or lying out in the sun on a lounge chair. You may think you're relaxed, but your shoulder muscles may still be tense or your neck feel tight—and you're so accustomed to it that the discomfort doesn't register at a conscious level. Meanwhile, your mind is still running a mile a minute, calculating unpaid bills or the work piling up at the office.

True relaxation is a physiologically powerful art that can easily be mastered. In this chapter I'll teach you to elicit "the relaxation response," a term coined by the relaxation researcher Herbert Benson, M.D., author of *Timeless Healing* and president of the Mind/Body Medical Institute at the Harvard-affiliated Beth Israel Deaconess Medical Center.

The relaxation response counteracts the harmful effects of sustained stress, the ultimate saboteur of health. Stress kills. How? Stress triggers the fight-or-flight response: Your adrenal glands churn out the stress hormone adrenaline, which quickens your heart rate and raises your blood pressure. This hormone can help you adapt very quickly to challenging or dangerous situations. But when stress persists over prolonged periods of time, elevated levels of another stress hormone, cortisol, can cause obesity, sexual dysfunction, memory problems, reduced immunity, and depression.

Chronic stress can also make your adrenal glands malfunction, so they cannot respond properly on a day-to-day basis. This can lower your already depleted energy levels, as well as your ability to cope with sudden stress. Long-term stress can also dampen your sex drive by shifting the resources of the adrenal glands away from production of the sex hormone precursor DHEA and toward the other adrenal hormones necessary for individual survival (such as cortisol). Stress actually intensifies your craving for sweets. Stress can affect your memory by being toxic to one set of memory cells in the brain, called the hippocampus. The hippocampus, shown to shrink in depression, returns to normal size after successful treatment of depression. *Persistent stressful life situations can counteract the beneficial effects of antidepressants and prevent a total recovery from your depression or medical condition.*

Numerous studies have documented the multiple physical and mental benefits of relaxation and Transcendental Meditation, from reduced blood pressure to reduced depression. The relaxation response is a tranquil state that works in opposition to the fight-or-flight response by lowering your blood pressure and decreasing your heart rate and breathing rate. It also boosts your brain's production of endorphins to make you feel calm and happy. In over two decades of research Benson and his colleagues have determined that getting your body into a relaxed state has a host of health benefits, from lowering your risk of heart disease to curing insomnia and restoring a happier outlook on your life. Getting your body into a relaxed state has another benefit: It can help keep your blood-sugar level on an even keel to reduce sugar cravings, a common side effect of antidepressants. Relaxation keeps cortisol levels down in the normal range; *high cortisol levels promote high blood sugar and high insulin levels, which cause sugar cravings, weight gain, and multiple diseases.*

Other researchers have also found that various relaxation techniques can stabilize mood swings and ease the blues, amplifying the effects of antidepressants. One study of thirty patients who were taking antidepressants for depression found that those who regularly practiced relaxation techniques experienced significant improvements in their moods compared with those who were not employing the techniques. Another study of patients with chronic pain found that those who practiced Transcendental Meditation experienced a major improvement in their pain symptoms, moods, and body image compared with those who took standard pain medications.

I recall a patient who suffered from chronic back pain after a fall. Tony, a real estate guru, was immobilized by intractable back pain and quickly became depressed. As a result of his fear of being permanently incapacitated, his pain and depression worsened, and Tony could not sleep at night. He would eat one or two bowls of cereal at 3:00 A.M. His weight had quickly gone up by over seventy pounds before I first saw him. Tony's worst fears had become reality—as so often happens when we focus obsessively on our fears. In addition to prescribing antidepressant medication for both his pain and his depression, I taught Tony relaxation techniques, which dramatically increased his ability to tolerate the pain. His sleep improved, his tension was reduced, and, astoundingly, he was able to lose all the weight he'd gained and throw away his cane. I remember how thrilled I was the first time I saw him walk into my office without his cane. (Tony was so grateful that he gave me a real estate tip!)

RELAXATION TECHNIQUES

Find one of the techniques detailed in this section that you can do for twenty minutes a day to elicit the relaxation response. The ideal activity combines physical and mental relaxation. While the goal of aerobic exercise is to boost your pulse rate and break a sweat, the goal of the relaxation response is to lower your pulse, breathing, and blood pressure, and to change your brain wave activity. You want to slow your breathing and heart rate and brush aside any mental distractions. Various means can elicit the relaxation response. Try a variety of techniques to break up your routine or pick the one that works best for you.

Note: You need to pick a time of day to relax when you can be free from distractions—when you can let the answering machine pick up and your kids are out of the house or asleep.

BENSON'S RELAXATION RESPONSE

First, sit comfortably in a chair or on the floor, and pick a focus word or short phrase that's firmly rooted in your personal belief system. Protestants could use "The Lord is my shepherd," Jews "Shema Yisroel," and so on, and nonreligious people "Nature heals" or any other phrase that has meaning for you. Close your eyes, and relax your muscles. Now, breathe slowly and naturally, repeating your focus word or phrase silently as you exhale.

Throughout, assume a passive attitude. Don't worry about whether you're performing the technique correctly. When other thoughts come, simply let them pass through you unacknowledged. Imagine your mind as a blank blackboard, and any time stray thoughts appear on the board, simply erase them and gently return to your repetition. Continue for fifteen to twenty minutes. You may open your eyes to check the time, but don't use an alarm. (The sounding of the alarm can be jarring and disrupt your relaxation.) When you finish, sit quietly for a minute or so, at first with your eyes closed and later with your eyes open. Then, remain seated for one or two minutes, stretch, and get up slowly.

PROGRESSIVE MUSCLE RELAXATION

Sit in a comfortable chair with back and head support, or lie on a lightly cushioned mat on the floor. (A bed is too soft, and in bed you're likely to fall asleep.) Tense each of your major muscle groups one at a time; inhale and slowly exhale as you release the tensed muscle group. Begin with your face, by wrinkling your forehead and shutting your eyes as tight as you can. Exhale and release. With each tensing-relaxing, imagine yourself floating deeper and deeper into the chair. Next, tense your neck and shoulders by drawing your shoulders up into a shrug. Exhale and release. Again, notice yourself floating deeper and deeper still into the chair, letting gravity pull you down. Work your way down to your arms and hands; press your palms together with your elbows pointing outward and push as hard as you can.

Exhale and release. Contract your stomach. Exhale and release. Arch your back and release. Now tense your hips and buttocks, pressing your legs and heels against the surface beneath you. Exhale and release. Point and flex your toes and release.

Next, tense all your muscles at once. Then take a deep breath, hold it, and exhale slowly as you relax the muscles, letting go of the tension. Feel your body at rest, floating deeper and deeper into the chair, and enjoy this state of relaxation for several minutes. If you prefer you can purchase or create an audiotape for yourself, guiding you through the various muscle groups. If you do this, speak slowly and allow yourself to relax, even as you make the tape. One advantage of a tape is that it allows you to be in a more passive state, where you simply follow directions and do not have to think.

MEDITATION

The focused awareness that comes with meditation can help you experience the transcendental interconnectedness of all living things. Or it can simply benefit you by lowering your blood pressure and respiration rate. Sit comfortably in a dignified position, with your head, neck, and back erect but not stiff. You can sit in a straight-backed chair or cross-legged on the floor. Choose a single object of focus, like your breathing or a portion of a prayer. Concentrate on the qualities of that object—the sounds, sensations, and thoughts—as they enter your awareness. Continue this for twenty minutes.

You can also practice meditation in a natural setting. A patient of mine named Sharon meditates outside to balance the stress of raising three young children. Every morning Sharon goes to her backyard deck and watches the sun rise while focusing on her breathing. "It's a time of peace and quiet," she says, "and I find it's a great way to ease myself into the day." Appreciating the beauty of nature allows you to transcend your own problems and reminds you of how vast the world really is. You can meditate while gazing up at the stars, the clouds, or the rippling surface of a pond. You may find that a meditation ritual strengthens your connection to God. Perhaps you have a special place—a church, synagogue, temple, or mosque, or even a meditation space in your home or garden—where you can sit in prayerful meditation.

MOVING MEDITATION

Joe, who is taking antidepressants after a diagnosis of cancer sent him into a depression, uses his relaxation time as a way to connect with his wife. "Every evening, no matter what the weather, we take a walk outside together holding hands," Joe says. "We have a policy that we don't discuss our problems or even talk during our relaxation walks. I usually focus on the sound of our feet hitting the pavement." Another patient of mine named Sally spends every afternoon rowing on a lake in a boat that she built herself. "I take my cat," she says, "and away we glide. No matter how stressed I am, the minute I climb into my boat, I immediately relax and clear my mind of any tension."

Both of these patients relax through what I call moving meditation. The idea is to move with mindful or even prayerful intentions. Remember to keep focused on the movement of your legs, the swinging rhythm of your arms, or the sound of your breath, while letting your mind drift away from any stress or tension.

YOGA

Yoga evokes a sense of serenity and what yoga experts refer to as mindfulness, a meditative focusing on the present moment. Many of my patients use yoga as a relaxation technique. Move through the various poses slowly and mindfully to get the benefit of relaxation.

RELAXATION QUICKIE

When you are stressed and feel yourself becoming tense, you may not be able to take a twenty-minute relaxation break. In these situations you can use a quick and effective relaxation technique developed by Dr. Christiane Northrup. Press your hand over your heart and close your eyes. While breathing deeply, recall someone or something you feel unconditional love for—a person, a place, even a song. Inhabit that loving feeling for a good moment or so. Open your eyes and take a deep breath.

Try it right now, before you read the next paragraph.

As you can see, all of these relaxation techniques are similar. Their main objective is to help you simply slow down enough, and release enough, to bring your consciousness back into focus, and back to the natural balance your body and psyche rediscover whenever stress is reduced. It doesn't take very long, but the benefits of relaxation can last the rest of the day. *Done routinely, relaxation has been shown to normalize adrenal hormone imbalances.*

REINTRODUCE PLAY INTO YOUR LIFE

Play is a fundamental way to reconnect with pleasure. It is an innate human activity that emerges during the first few months of life, when infants begin to laugh at a game of peekaboo. Children are the masters of play. They invoke their spirits and imaginations to conjure up a pirate ship out of a couch or a three-ring circus out of a tent of blankets and a few stuffed animals. And children will do anything for a laugh. Child's play takes many forms (laughter, wrestling, tickling, creation, imitation, and so on) and is essential to cognitive and motor development, stress reduction, and emotional connection to others.

One of the hallmarks of children's play is how effortlessly they can enter it. As we grow into adulthood we lose touch with our play instinct. This is partially a neurological development and partially a by-product of socialization. Play is gradually marginalized in our adult lives, to the point where daydreaming, humor, and sex are virtually our only remaining arenas of sanctioned play. Too often we get lazy and turn to artificial chemical inducers of pleasure, like drinking alcohol, smoking cigarettes, or biting into a tasty chocolate bar. Although these may give us a momentary sensation of pleasure, in the long run they debilitate our bodies, emotions, and spirits.

Play is any activity that's fun. Put another way, it's an intrinsically motivated activity, meaning that play is its own reward. No one is paying you or in any way rewarding you for it. (So a professional football player is only really "playing" in those moments when he's not thinking about his career or his upcoming contract renewal. Similarly, your weekly squash game stops being play the moment it becomes a social obligation.)

Play is whatever turns you on: taking a thrilling sled ride down a snowy hill or jumping off the swings in midair at the park. Play is laughing at your spouse's joke or tickling a baby's tummy. Play is riding the waves with your friends at the beach or creating a sand castle on the shore. Play is the leavener of life, and one of its most natural and effective painkillers. It will help you regain the carefree spirit you lost to adulthood or depression, and it pays immediate dividends in the form of pleasure. Some adults have a more natural aptitude for play than others—we all know, and envy, innately playful people—but I believe that we can all recapture some measure of the playfulness we had as children.

Researchers are discovering that play builds denser webs of neural connections and that this reserve of brainpower can be crucial for retaining memory and mental sharpness as we age. Play should involve some sense of novelty to stimulate your pleasure centers and increase your involvement. Your brain is wired to respond to novelty, and the fresher the activity, the more engaged you become. Researchers at the University of California at Berkeley found that rats allowed to play with toys learned to traverse mazes more quickly and had significantly thicker cerebral cortexes than rats who did not play. Once the toys were taken away from the rats, their cerebral cortexes shrank back to normal size.

Play can be a solitary activity, although you may find you get more of a brain boost and feel more exhilarated when you're playing with someone else. And sharing a smile or a laugh with a friend or stranger will strengthen emotional connections that may have been severed when you were depressed or ill. Play is one of the first steps toward developing or repairing an intimate relationship.

LAUGHTER AS A TONIC FOR DEPRESSION

Humor is a therapeutic form of verbal play. My most enduring and fond memories of childhood and family are all centered on humor, a facility with which we have all been blessed. Both in my personal life and in my psychiatric practice, I've come to appreciate humor as a creative and healing force.

People who are stressed or depressed often lose their ability to laugh or find situations humorous. Everything becomes serious, and thinking becomes negatively charged on every level. This is partially because depression reduces the blood flow to those regions of your brain that are able to make associations between incongruous concepts that are normally not connected. For instance, in an episode of *Seinfeld,* Kramer decided to invent the man-ssiere, a bra for men. To appreciate the humor of this premise, your brain's cortex (the region of higher thought processes) needs to link quickly two previously unconnected concepts, which don't belong in the same word: bras for men.

Using positron-emission tomography (PET), researchers have been able to document a decreased blood flow to the cortex in the brains of depressed patients. Studies have also shown that antidepressants can restore the blood flow to the cortex, so you can once again experience the lighter side of life. And the more you laugh, the more you activate the dopamine pleasure pathways that became dormant when you were depressed. Laughter works its magic by triggering your brain's release of a multitude of pleasure-enhancing chemicals; dopamine activity increases in parts of your limbic system—a key emotional center in your brain—with feelings of exhilaration and happiness, while endorphins can actually numb physical and emotional pain. In fact, research has found that the very act of forming a smile can make you feel relaxed and happy by transmitting nerve impulses from the facial muscles to your brain to tilt your neurochemical balance toward happiness.

Laughter has another benefit: It can provide an immediate release from built-up tension—much in the way that relaxation exercises can. Do you ever remember laughing uncontrollably when, according to authority figures, you were supposed to be serious (in class, or even at a funeral)? The more you were supposed to ignore the subject, the more you wanted to laugh! Charles Darwin viewed laughter as a means of discharging surplus tension. He believed that laughter restores equilibrium and stimulates circulation to create a sense of well-being. Several studies suggest that laughter can help alleviate phobias and other anxiety disorders and reduce pain, and some psychologists use it as a form of psychotherapy. In the movie *Patch Adams,* Robin Williams portrays a real-life doctor who wears clown makeup and a red, bulbous nose to entertain his patients. "Humor is the antidote to all ills" is a phrase he often repeats.

I worked with a patient named Barbara who was suffering from depression. Antidepressants weren't working fully to alleviate her fears of dying young. At every therapy session this thirty-five-year-old single

mother discussed her fears in detail, though she intellectually understood them to be groundless. "Maybe I'll get killed in a car crash or
develop some terminal form of cancer," Barbara said. "I can't envision
myself as a grandmother. In fact, I know I'm never going to live to see
my grandchildren and probably won't see my own children grow up."
She told me that she couldn't stop worrying about how her two young
children would manage without her. "I don't have a life," she complained. "I'm just existing."

I said to her, "Existing? You're not even existing. You've already
sentenced yourself to death. I bet you've hired an undertaker and
picked out a nice black casket with red velvet lining. I wouldn't be surprised if you'd hired your brother's party planner to arrange your
funeral!" Barbara laughed and began to realize that maybe she could
find a way to redirect her energies to enjoying life rather than preparing for death.

We began to focus on fun things she could plan with her children. She started taking them to amusement parks and indoor play
centers. "I crawl through the tunnels and go on the roller coasters with
them. I've actually been having fun. I can't believe that I forgot what
fun felt like."

Although I don't go to the extreme of dressing as a clown for my
patients (yet), or claiming laughter will cure all ills, I do incorporate
playfulness and humor into the creative practice of medicine and help
my patients to see their problems in a humorous way, while acknowl-
edging their real-life dilemmas. Just as laughing over a meal improves
digestion, laughing improves our ability to digest life.

MY PRESCRIPTION FOR A PLAYFUL LIFE

Play, of course, needs to be somewhat spontaneous and cannot be
planned. You can't conjure up a laugh at will or schedule a tickle session with your kids. You can, however, *make the decision to interact more
playfully with others,* to give life to those quiet impulses that lurk in
everyone's funny bones, to pursue activities for the sheer purpose of having fun. At first you may be making a conscious effort to play, but before
long playing will become a natural instinct. This is what I suggest.

Get Small Doses of Play Throughout the Day

Weave play into the fabric of your life. Try some of the following, or make your own list. The more novel the activity, the more fun you'll have.

* Tickle someone you love.
* Joke with the people on the elevator.
* Play charades.
* Grab a joke book and tell one joke a day.
* Roll around on the floor with a pet or a child. Engage in a little free play.
* Grab a board game or deck of cards. The great thing about games is that they are fresh and new every time you play.
* Spend a few minutes doodling on a piece of paper with a friend. Choose a theme: dream houses, the perfect gift, your boss. Compare your renderings. (I just went to lunch with my staff and suggested we all draw what we were thinking. We got a few good laughs out of that!)
* Have fun with the seasons. Have a snowball fight; build a snowman; jump in a pile of leaves; run around under a lawn sprinkler; take a walk in the rain.
* Into scavenger hunts? Get a few friends together and hit a local park or beach.
* Go to a comedy club or see a funny movie with a friend or loved one.
* Scan the weekend section of your paper and find at least one thing to do that is totally out of character for you—whether it's going to the circus or browsing at an antiques fair.
* Surprise your family by serving them breakfast for dinner and dinner for breakfast.
* Play a practical joke (but do no harm!).

Develop a Playful Passion

Find an activity that intrinsically motivates you and gives you pleasure. Perhaps you want to create a thing of beauty by knitting, sculpting, or painting. Maybe you enjoy stamp collecting. Make a commitment to take up a pleasurable activity that normally gets squeezed out of everyday life. It should be something that is preceded by the phrase "I've always wanted to learn…" or "I used to love to…" But remember, do not take the activity too seriously. Inject it with humor.

I filled in this blank for myself a few years ago and decided to take up scuba diving. As a child I used to dream about visiting other planets, becoming an astronaut. I took a course in scuba diving and planned a vacation around it. I found that being underwater was as close to visiting another world as anyone on this planet can get. The colors are more vibrant than one can imagine, one is nearly weightless, and the view is beyond description. I rented a camera and took some pictures underwater, including some very funny ones (I thought) of me feeding Cheez Whiz to the fish.

Getting passionate about fun can give you regular doses of joy in your everyday life. What's more, it can help you live longer. Researchers have found that pursuing playful passions can boost your immune system, which helps ward off diseases from colds to cancer.

Join a Sports League

A fifty-year-old female patient of mine joined a softball league and plays with teenagers. Joining a soccer, baseball, touch football, or other sports league gives you a double benefit: You get your exercise and play wrapped in one. Resist the temptation for play to become competitive and enjoy the camaraderie instead.

Revisit Your Childhood

I knew a sixty-five-year-old woman who had played the violin as a child and decided to go back to it. Go back to the piano or guitar that you haven't touched in years. Reclaim all those ribbons you won in horseback riding.

SPIRITUAL RENEWAL

In *God in Search of Man* (a truly inspirational book I would recommend to readers of all faiths), Abraham J. Heschel wrote:

> *Away from the immense, cloistered in our own concepts,*
> *we may scorn and revile everything.*
> *But standing between heaven and earth, we are silenced.*

Depression is like being trapped in an internal hell, "cloistered in our own concepts." Antidepressants can elevate us back to the terrestrial plane, where our despair is silenced—or at least muted. But looking upward and outward—for instance, at the star-studded sky on a clear night—revives our sense of awe and perspective.

One of the few silver linings in the dark cloud of depression is that it makes you confront the tough questions that many people avoid. Is there any meaning to life? Does God, or any higher power or spiritual dimension, exist? Depression no doubt tested your faith in life and in yourself. Like the biblical Job, you may have had to look within your deepest self—into your soul—to keep from falling totally into the abyss.

And since you survived, you were probably able to locate and cling to some particle of faith or belief. I encourage you to build on whatever piece of faith you've salvaged from your encounter with depression and use it to renew your spiritual life. In the wake of depression it's easy to surrender to cynicism. But if you want a life that includes joy, you cannot allow yourself to be ruled by doubt. I'm not suggesting that you overrule doubt—just don't let it run your life. One of Heschel's central tenets is that faith is a relative matter; we all navigate somewhere between total faith and total disbelief. Heschel advises that we work with our "ball of doubt" to journey toward faith.

When I talk about faith, I'm not referring to any particular religion or organized faith. But no matter how battered you may have been by depression, resuming life is impossible without faith in something. The French philosopher René Descartes applied his intellectual skepticism to the task of reducing his faith to its smallest component. His conclusion: "I think, therefore I am." For Descartes, the ability to think was the one truth that he could not doubt. Buddha reduced his faith to Four Noble Truths, the first being that everything is in a state of continual change. The Golden Rule—Do unto others as you would have them do unto you—is another example of an article of faith reduced to its barest, purest form. The poet John Keats proclaimed:

> *Beauty is truth, truth beauty—that is all*
> *ye know on earth, and all ye need to know.*

I encourage you to find and cleave to your own article of faith—not for any moral reason, but because it's good for you. The idea that believing in God or a higher power is good for your health has been confirmed by 75 percent of the more than three hundred studies conducted on healing and religion. Deeply religious people of all faiths seem to benefit in several areas: less substance abuse, lower rates of depression and anxiety, enhanced quality of life, and longer life expectancy. Even if you're living a secular life, simply acting in accordance with your values can improve your health. In a 1996 study of women aged thirty-five to eighty, researchers at Salem College in Winston-Salem, North Carolina, found that living according to their beliefs and relying on their faith in those belief systems in times of stress reduced high blood pressure and helped the women feel less stressed overall.

No one can outline a spiritual path for you to follow in any more than a general sense (pursue your grandest vision of yourself, cultivate the best that's within you). You are your own best guide. What I can do is encourage you to *recognize and explore your own path* and share the experiences of a few of my patients. Their journeys may inspire your own.

JENNIE'S PATH

Jennie, a twenty-seven-year-old singer, was severely depressed when I first met her. Her college education never quite got off the ground. Her depression had been rearing its head intermittently since her adolescence, when her mother died and her life was thrown into chaos. Despite a very loving and supportive father, she could not find her direction in life. Jennie contemplated suicide on several occasions but would not give it serious thought because she could not hurt her father. After being on lithium and Wellbutrin for two years, Jennie was finally trusting her sense of emotional stability, but she still lacked direction.

During one session I asked Jennie when she was happiest in her life. Her answer was quick and to the point: "I remember being in a musical in eighth grade. I sang two songs and was never happier than those weeks and months of practice and performance." I asked why that experience was so satisfying. Her reply surprised me. "Aside from being the center of attention, what I really loved was being able to convey the warm and loving emotions of the songs to the audience. The mixture of voice, lyrics, and instruments conveys this in a way no other medium can, as far as I'm concerned. I feel so intimately connected to the audience, as if I'm serenading my lover."

Jennie dismissed the notion of singing professionally because she didn't feel talented enough to be successful. I encouraged her, and encouraged her father to support her if that was her best vision of herself. Jennie slowly geared herself up by taking some voice lessons, to the point that she could audition for a part. Despite not getting chosen on her first round of auditions, she prevailed and eventually was cast in a local musical.

Alan's Path

Religion is a tool that can enhance your spirituality by strengthening your connection to a higher being. If religion is practiced effectively, it can increase respect and compassion for all people. It can also provide a supportive community and a way to incorporate a spiritual ritual into your life.

Alan, a thirty-nine-year-old businessman, was raised in a nonobservant Jewish home. He loved his wife, child, parents, and brother and two sisters but felt alone and depressed. He felt something was missing, but he didn't know what it was. Alan had achieved his professional goals at a relatively young age, and he wondered if this was all there was.

His doctor put him on Zoloft, which reduced the nagging anxiety and depression, and allowed him to shelve the paralyzing existential questions. However, the Zoloft left him with sexual side effects and a twenty-pound weight gain. Alan came to me for a second opinion, wondering whether he was on the right medication.

As we reviewed his life story, it became clear that Alan had had a pattern of low-grade depression since the middle years of high school. His family history also pointed to chronic depression. As part of the history taking, I delved into Alan's spiritual life, which was largely nonexistent, despite the larger questions he had grappled with. When I told Alan that some of the best minds of the century have concluded that all of life's problems ultimately come down to spiritual questions, he was relieved, because he had been embarrassed to raise the issue with anyone in his family. Several of his family members had been killed in the Holocaust, and as a result any belief in God or religion was scoffed at.

Alan began quietly to explore his Jewish heritage, studied the Holocaust, and attended synagogue. His biggest hurdle was coming to terms with man's inhumanity to man, and God's role in that. After he joined a liberal Reform synagogue and participated in Bible study groups, his life felt much more rounded out and fulfilling. He hasn't resolved his biggest questions of faith, but he's engaged in active inquiry in the company of others, and for Alan that's made a huge difference.

MONA'S PATH

Even if you lead a secular life, you can create spiritual rituals. The key is to find a way to unify yourself with the world at large by cultivating an awareness of the moment, the now. There are countless vehicles for spiritual connection: music, nature, poetry, or sports.

Mona discovered that her path to spiritual connection lay in gardening. Having gone through two marriages and two careers (as a stockbroker and a psychotherapist), Mona was depressed. She felt like a complete failure, and being childless added to her loneliness. Mona had had several episodes of depression in her adult years, and now, at age fifty-two, she felt more depressed than ever.

Mona responded quite well to Luvox and was more cheerful within weeks. She embarked on my program and improved her nutrition, regulated her hormones, and started exercising regularly. There was no question that Mona was better, but there was also no question that Mona did not yet have a life—because she had no joy.

I asked her my well-worn question: "Mona, when were you happiest in your life?" As it turned out, Mona was not happiest when she was with a man, or when she was selling stocks or doing psychotherapy. Mona was always her happiest when she was in her garden. She told me, "The beauty of flowers makes me understand that there must be a greater power. This kind of beauty cannot be an accident. It just cannot be. When I remember this, I feel calm, and I know there is some purpose to our lives. And beauty is an important part of it."

With encouragement from me to follow her passion, Mona took

courses in landscape design and has started her own business. She believes that at this point in her life bringing beauty into the foreground of people's awareness is her main purpose, and she is happier than she has been in years.

SUMMING UP

Renewing your spiritual life is a central component of the Antidepressant Survival Program. If you're not depressed anymore but still feel rudderless, if you aren't in despair anymore but feel marooned on an island of doubt, my best advice is to get a spiritual life. Find what's most meaningful to you, plant it in the ground, and water it.

My favorite children's book is a simple and profound tale of faith by Ruth Krauss called *The Carrot Seed*. It begins, "A little boy planted a carrot seed." Everyone in his life (his mother, his father, and his older brother) assured him, "It won't come up." Undaunted, the little boy watered the seed and pulled up the weeds around it. "But nothing came up." So the little boy kept watering and weeding. "And then, one day, a carrot came up just as the little boy had known it would."

The final picture in the book shows the little boy pushing a wheelbarrow with an enormous carrot in it, his face set with determination, direction, and purpose.

Plant your own carrot seed. Water it with patience, and you will reap the harvest. And answer the question for yourself: *"When was I happiest in my life?"*

The Medical Prescription

Forging a Partnership with Your Doctor

* * *

The Hormone Connection

* * *

Gut Reactions

* * *

Reclaiming a Healthy Sex Drive

THIS SECTION BEGINS the part of the Antidepressant Survival Program that I call the Medical Prescription. In treating well over fifteen hundred patients with antidepressants, I've compiled a streamlined list of hidden medical conditions that can aggravate or even cause the side effects you may be experiencing. They can also interfere with the therapeutic effects of antidepressants by hindering your normal metabolic function.

These conditions can cause weight gain, drain your vitality, and destroy your sex life. The medical conditions most commonly associated with antidepressant use fall into three major categories: hormone imbalances, gut reactions, and sexual malfunctions. Although the Fundamentals part of my program can restore many of the physiological imbalances caused by antidepressants, it can't provide a cure for every problem. *The good news is that the vast majority of these conditions can be cured or managed with straightforward, noninvasive treatments.*

A wide range of medical problems—from adrenal system abnormalities to zinc deficiency—cause symptoms that mimic the side effects of antidepressants. They also may cause or contribute to depressed moods, which curtail the benefits of the antidepressants. Some of these problems actually result from the use of antidepressants. These are what I call the casualties of antidepressants. In a war waged with antidepressants, innocent bystanders—like your thyroid gland or your sex organs—may be wounded. As the antidepressants normalize your moods or relieve the pain of a debilitating medical condition, these body systems can shift off balance, causing new problems or pushing old, undiagnosed problems into the foreground. As do the majority of my patients, you may find that the Medical Prescription is a vital complement to the Fundamentals.

Although the Medical Prescription is incorporated into the final chapters of this book, I usually begin this diagnostic work-up at the initial appointment with a new patient. Right after our first handshake, I dive into my questions. They consist of the standard psychiatric evaluation (a history of the problem, current stressors, any previous psychiatric history, a detailed three-generation family history, a personal history, and a mental status exam) as well as an evaluation of the various systems that may be involved in promoting side effects or symptoms (hormonal, diet and nutrition, gastrointestinal, immune function, lifestyle, and so on) and a limited physical examination. At the close of the visit, I can summarize the problems and systems I suspect are involved and order a series of diagnostic tests to get an accurate reading on the systems of the body that could be out of balance. I then explain the concepts of my program and discuss the benefits of healthy lifestyle changes. If a patient is ready to proceed with the program, I get him or her started: "Before you come in for your follow-up, I'm giving you an assignment; first do the Jump Start and then move on to the nutrition plan and exercise program."

We schedule a follow-up appointment for about a month later to discuss the test results and necessary treatments. During the next appointment I check to see if there has been any decrease in side effects or enhanced efficacy of the medication. *Some of my patients with hormone irregularities or other medical conditions find that they can alleviate these problems simply by following the Fundamentals!* The vast majority get significant benefit from the Fundamentals; however, they also need some type of medical intervention in addition to the lifestyle changes.

Just as I work closely with my patients, the Medical Prescription requires you to consult closely with your own doctor. In each chapter I have inserted sections called Note to Your Doctor, in which I indicate the reasons for my recommendations and give specific guidance on tests and treatments. These notes may read to you like a lot of technical jargon. Ask your doctor to explain them if you want to learn more about your specific medical condition.

I'd like you to schedule an appointment to see your doctor during the first few weeks that you're on the program. Then take the self-evaluation quizzes that I've included in each of the next three chapters to see if you have signs of a hidden medical condition that requires treatment. Your doctor will take a more complete medical history and order the appropriate diagnostic tests. You will then need to have a follow-up appointment about four to six weeks later to go over the test results and discuss any treatments you might need. You might also want to enlist your therapist's help in supporting you on the program. If you're not in therapy, a trusted friend, family member, or clergyperson can serve in this support role.

CHAPTER SEVEN

Forging a Partnership for Healing with Your Doctor

Traps to Avoid, Questions to Ask, Tools to Share

* * *

IF YOU'RE ON ANTIDEPRESSANT medication, you already have a relationship with a doctor. He or she might be a psychiatrist, an internist, a gynecologist, or a family practitioner. You may think of this person as your friend, your adversary, or a bureaucrat of the medical care system, depending on the kinds of experiences you've shared—as well as the experiences you've had with other doctors or authority figures. Regardless, you've probably invested a lot of time and money in this relationship, so it's in your interest to make it as productive as you possibly can.

As you can probably tell, I'm trying to change the way many doctors use antidepressant medications. But my goal isn't to bash doctors. Neither do I want to replace your doctor; no book can give you the kind of personal attention and care that a doctor can. Rather, I hope this book and my program can build a bridge between you and your doctor. I want to help you forge a specific kind of relationship with your physician—a relationship based on trust, communication, cooperation, and pragmatism. Think of your doctor as your *partner* in healing.

What exactly do I mean by *partner*? Partners in any relationship, by definition, have common goals. In addition, effective partnerships are characterized by each individual bringing his or her unique strengths, history, and perspective to bear on those goals. When these different perspectives are respected and valued—rather than allowed to become a source of contention—the partnership benefits from increased flexibility and resources. When patients and their doctors approach each other with mutual respect and a shared sense of purpose, the patients are the ultimate beneficiaries.

In the training seminars I conduct for psychiatrists and other mental health professionals, I'm always favorably impressed by their eagerness to acquire the tools to help their patients overcome side effects and amplify benefits of their medications. Wherever I speak or teach these days, I hear a consensus building among doctors that side effects are pandemic among their patients on antidepressants. These doctors are concerned and want to learn how to treat them. And I'm consistently impressed by the enthusiasm and open-mindedness of the psychiatrists in training (in the classes on affective disorders and psychoendocrinology I teach at Georgetown University Hospital).

Nevertheless, it takes two to form a partnership. If your current doctor won't meet you halfway, you need to find one who will. In Appendix One, I'll guide you to sources that can help you find doctors who are knowledgeable about psychopharmacology and receptive to an integrative treatment approach.

The Medical Prescription will give you and your doctor hands-on tools for building your partnership. Your doctor doesn't have to be a specialist in endocrinology or psychopharmacology to help you succeed with the program. All that's required is an open mind, a willingness to learn, and an abiding concern for the best interest of the patient (that's you!). In these chapters I provide the directions the two of you will need to complete the medical sections of the program. Other parts you can do on your own—but it's a good idea to include your doctor in these parts too, since they're all interconnected and directly related to getting the most therapeutic results from your medications. Remember, it's a partnership; don't keep your partner in the dark.

THE DOCTOR-PATIENT COVENANT

People tend to have complicated relationships with their doctors—for some obvious and not-so-obvious reasons. Since you're entrusting your doctor with your health and well-being, this relationship is clearly a higher-stakes transaction than your relationship with your attorney or accountant. And since you're the one who's "sick" and your doctor is the putative healer—or at least the medical expert—it's difficult to feel like an equal partner. It is not surprising, then, that many people experience childlike feelings of dependency, inadequacy, and helplessness with their doctors, and that these emotions are often expressed along a wide spectrum, ranging from love and devotion to passivity, antagonism, or even hate.

For their part, some doctors enjoy their status and are loath to grant equality to their patients. They've devoted years—often decades—to their medical education and training. It's not easy for them to have their knowledge questioned by their patients. They sometimes forget that *you, the patient, are the one with firsthand knowledge of the problem they are trying to solve,* as well as the understanding of how that problem fits in with the rest of your life. You are the one living with it twenty-four hours a day, seven days a week. *You are the expert witness of your own condition.*

Despite their seeming position of power, knowledge, and control, many doctors become insecure in the face of difficult cases, such as depression and the side effects of medication. Doctors are results-oriented people who want and are expected to have all the answers. When they can't solve a problem or come up with definitive answers, some doctors may simply give up—"I can't help you, and I don't know who can. There is nothing more I can do"—while others may become defensive, since they are not inclined to accept failures graciously—"Look, I've done all I can do. If you're unsatisfied, find someone else to work with."

You may be one of the many patients on antidepressants who reach an impasse with their doctors. Dissatisfied with the "half a life" remedy of partial response to antidepressants and their associated side effects, you still may not feel entitled to demand help from your physician. And if you do stand up for yourself, you may be met with ignorance, in the true sense of the word, or defensiveness. Your doctor may dismiss your complaints as trivial compared with depression—or he or she may simply not be sophisticated enough about psychopharmacology, nutrition, endocrinology, immunology, neurology, or gastrointestinal function to offer useful advice.

I think of the relationship between doctors and their patients as a sacred covenant. As in any covenant, both parties have rights and responsibilities. Each of you plays a vital role: your doctor supplying essential medical experience and access to prescriptive medicine and testing, you agreeing to communicate candid, accurate information on your symptoms and condition, then faithfully following through on your mutually agreed treatment plan.

Like any covenant, this one needs to be based on trust, communication, and mutual respect. Sounds simple enough, but it's a tall order. Speaking as a doctor who's had to work at accepting his patients as equals and communicating with them, let me try to give you some insight into how we make doctors. This should help you take the first steps toward forging an optimal partnership with your doctor.

THE TRAINING AND MISTRAINING OF DOCTORS

Contrary to popular opinion, the vast majority of doctors are initially motivated by compassion, not financial gain, when they enter the medical profession. But they're human—a condition that a lot of doctors and patients collude in obscuring. And the human failings of many doctors are exacerbated by their "trial by fire" medical education and training.

Let me begin by telling you a few things about my own training, which was typical of what most young doctors went through in the 1970s. Frankly, when I began my career in medicine, I did not know how to care for my patients. It wasn't that I was unconcerned or lazy or cynical. My difficulty in those early days, rather, arose from two central facts about being a doctor. First, I had serious anxiety about being able to master all the medical knowledge I was responsible for—I didn't want to harm anyone. And, second, the medical establishment generally did not place a high premium on relating to the patient as a whole person.

Put bluntly, caring for the patient's emotional needs was seen as irrelevant—*treating the disease was everything.* Understanding the patient's personal history and relationships was seen as "soft" medicine and virtually irrelevant to the cure. We were taught to focus all our attention on diagnosing and treating the patient's illness and decoding the results of laboratory tests. The patient was merely a source of information. This information was gleaned either physically, by observing signs of illness, or verbally, as symptoms described by the patient. During my medical school years I rarely had a meaningful conversation with a patient. In fact, shocking and embarrassing as it is to me now, it never even occurred to me that I should get to know the person with the disease—nor were there any models of such behavior in the nonpsychiatric world of "real doctors."

My training as an intern was an intense, grueling routine. I made my hurried hospital rounds, looking at the lab reports for all the patients, stopping in to see them, examining the ailing body parts or functions, eliciting any new complaints—"How's your liver today, Mrs. Smith?" I would order more tests, if needed, change orders for the nurses, and check lab results as they came in, then order more tests for the night and morning when necessary. Every other night I was on call, meaning that at the end of the day all the other physicians signed out their patients to me, telling me their general status and any potential problems. I could be responsible for as few as thirty patients or as many as there were in the entire hospital—a terrifying concept.

The night was spent in and out of the emergency room, evaluating people for admission, stabilizing the severely ill after admission, and sometimes attending to life-and-death emergencies. Rarely was there time for much sleep. Night rolled into day without distinction, a blur of donuts and coffee, and the routine started again. Fatigued and under constant stress, I prayed that I would not harm or kill anyone.

One night I was among the small handful of interns covering the entire hospital, and a patient who had had a recent stroke suffered a seizure, probably triggered by a second stroke. He was in his seventies, and I was unable to save him. His petite, white-haired wife sat in the waiting room, and now I had to deliver the news.

As gently as I could, I told the widow, "I'm sorry." I paused. "Your husband has died." Pause. "I—we tried."

I suppose she saw the pain on my face. She looked at me with such gentleness and warmth. Without a trace of anger, she touched my arm and said, "That's OK. I know you did your best." *She* was comforting *me*.

It bothered me deeply that my best hadn't been good enough. But more than that, it bothered me that, in an odd way, I had no feelings at all for this man—we'd never even spoken! I wish to this day that I'd cared enough to ask his wife about him—and, most of all, I wish I'd had the generosity to comfort her in her loss, rather than her having to comfort me.

That was how my life went for three hundred and sixty-five days. High levels of responsibility, not enough knowledge or experience, little sleep, and miserable nutrition. Doctors of internal medicine follow the same wearing routine for three years. It takes a toll.

The worst element of this system, however, is the deep effect it has on the young doctors' attitude toward patients. It breeds cynicism and dehumanization. To an intern stressed to the limit, patients become threatening on many levels. They mean more work. They may present potentially unsolvable medical problems. They may threaten total failure—in other words, death. At the very minimum they are a source of further sleep deprivation. Why must they always get sick at four in the morning!

Over the years, of course, many doctors are able to outgrow the trauma of this indoctrination, recovering the caring, humanitarian motives that brought them to med school in the first place. In my case, being trained as a psychiatrist during my residency, I was encouraged early on to listen—very carefully—to my patients. This aided my recovery from medical school and internship. And along the way I had several personal experiences with doctors that woke me up to the distant, patronizing attitude of some members of the medical profession. What I think of as the little tomato episode was one of the most vivid.

When I was thirty-four years old, married, and a father of three children, I was having digestive problems and gaining some unwanted weight. So I went to my physician for a checkup. "I notice that I can't tolerate dairy," I said. "I frequently get stomachaches and loose bowels. And I don't seem to be able to tolerate tomatoes—they drive me straight to the bathroom."

My doctor looked me up and down with a dismissive air and pronounced his conclusion: "Well, you don't look malnourished to me."

Period. End of discussion.

I felt embarrassed that I'd even brought up my complaints. I left the office feeling foolish. I'd received no help, no suggestions, no understanding. But this incident taught me an invaluable lesson in the art of caring—or, more properly, the consequences of not caring. I had to admit the truth—that I'd just been given a small dose of the callous treatment I and my fellow interns had unthinkingly dished out for years in the guise of medical care.

I'm telling you these war stories not because I want you to feel anger at the medical establishment or compassion for the hard life interns lead. Instead, I want you to understand a bit more about what it's like to walk in your doctor's shoes. It's all too easy these days to view your doctor as an adversary. Managed care encourages this feeling by putting pressure on doctors to provide less care. Lawyers encourage it by making a living on malpractice. And the medical establishment itself encourages ill feeling through its belief in the disease-centered, rather than patient-centered, treatment model.

You may well have encountered doctors who dismiss your side effects from antidepressants as trivial. While this might seem cold and uncaring on their part, it actually flows directly out of the way they were trained to evaluate the side effects of all medications. In medical school we learned to divide medication side effects into three categories: contraindications, serious side effects, and acceptable side effects.

Contraindications are side effects so serious that, given certain conditions, the drug must never be taken. For example, one must never take Demerol with an MAO-inhibitor antidepressant, because seizures will often result.

Serious side effects are those that the doctor and patient must be alert to and that may require discontinuation of the drug. For example, taking the mood stabilizer Tegretol may wipe out the bone marrow in a small percentage of patients. While this is a rare circumstance, the doctor and patient must keep a watchful eye out for such problems.

So-called *acceptable side effects* are those that are not life threatening and do not cause a risk of significant physical or mental harm.

In the normal course of events, when your doctor treats you successfully with an antidepressant, he or she remembers how you looked at your first appointment. If you complain about side effects, your doctor is likely to compare your "before" with your "after." If he or she feels satisfied there has been significant progress, the doctor will tend to minimize the importance of your side effects or partial improvement. After all, the reasoning goes, no one ever died for lack of a sex life, a trim figure, or an optimal level of energy. If you've gained significant weight, your doctor may not understand that it is your medication that has driven your appetite control and metabolism out of balance. He or she may conclude, instead, that weight control is an emotionally based problem for you to work out on your own—or, perhaps, that there are no alternatives to living with your drug's side effects or limited benefits.

And then there's the problem of managed care. Patients are understandably disgruntled by the bottom-line approach to medical care that seems to drive so many health plans. What you might not know is that doctors are just as unhappy about having bureaucrats telling them how to treat their patients. After years of training and professional experience, doctors are deeply disturbed that they are being told what and how much therapy they can administer, how much time they can spend with patients, and how much they'll be paid. The end result is to put more pressure on doctors to see more patients and spend less time and resources on them.

Despite these obstacles, you don't have to fall into the trap of viewing your doctor as your adversary. At the end of the day, the vast majority of doctors are genuinely caring people fully committed to helping their patients achieve good health. Few things make a doctor feel more satisfied than helping patients significantly improve their lives. Which is why forging a covenant of trust and communication with your doctor is an achievable goal.

YOUR BILL OF RIGHTS

A reciprocal relationship is one that involves both rights and responsibilities, both respect and accountability. In your relationship with your doctor, each of you has a different knowledge base. *You are the expert on what and how you are feeling and the facts of your life history.* Your doctor is the medical expert. In general, your doctor's foremost responsibility is to work toward the restoration of your health in a respectful manner, keeping up with the state of the art. In return, a doctor has the right to expect you to give honest information, to abide by your treatment plan, to interact as courteously and respectfully as your condition permits, and to behave responsibly when using his or her on-call emergency availability.

As a patient, you have the right to

* Be treated with respect and dignity
* Understand your doctor's recommendation—get answers to your questions
* Make your opinions and feelings heard
* Disagree
* Have a doctor whose primary concern, above all, is your health
* Get a consultation or a second opinion, or change doctors
* Make final decisions about your treatment—it is your health that is at stake

YOUR RESPONSIBILITIES

Like most doctors, I strive to do the best I can by each and every patient. But I am often surprised by how much my feelings about patients vary depending on how difficult or pleasant they are to deal with. And since I'm only human, those feelings can't help but affect my emotional (as opposed to merely professional) commitment to their successful treatment. The patients I most enjoy working with have a number of traits in common. They tend to be respectful of my skills and needs as their doctor. They are honest with me. They recognize that there are not always simple solutions to complex problems.

I believe that in a healthy patient-doctor relationship, the patient has certain responsibilities as well. These are actually responsibilities to your healing partnership with your doctor rather than to your doctor. Put another way, these are responsibilities to your own best medical interests.

In addition to paying your bills, you have a responsibility to:

* Be forthcoming and honest, even about embarrassing problems.
* Be prepared for your appointment, with questions clearly in mind or written out.
* Be reasonably aware of your symptoms and how they vary.
* Listen carefully and make sure you understand what your doctor says.
* Be aware of the demands on the doctor's time. This means prioritizing your concerns and keeping your appointment focused on relevant matters.
* Follow through on the agreed treatment plan. Do not make changes—especially medication changes—without consultation.
* Express appreciation for the doctor's efforts.
* Allow the doctor to be human.

TAKING YOUR DOCTOR'S TEMPERATURE

With these rights and responsibilities in mind, let's consider your working relationship with your doctor right now. There are three paramount issues to assess: communication, accessibility, and openness.

1. *Communication.* How well do you and your doctor communicate with each other? Do you feel uncomfortable or unwilling to discuss your problems, especially those that embarrass you, with your doctor? How much of this unwillingness is your responsibility? How much is caused by your doctor's manner? If your communication is not what it should be, how much improvement is realistically possible?

2. *Accessibility.* How available is your doctor? Do you have enough time during appointments to air your concerns and get clear responses? Do you feel confident that you can reach your doctor in an emergency or that he or she will respond to your urgent need for a telephone consultation?

3. *Openness.* Does your doctor seem open to new ideas, or does he or she act as if modern medicine has all the answers? (Some authorities estimate that as much as 80 percent of what we consider medical fact is altered every ten years, which also makes a very good case for a healthy dose of open-mindedness.) Does your doctor make an effort to keep up with current literature and the latest medical research? (You can partially answer these questions by learning how frequently your doctor teaches, writes papers and books, or attends working medical conferences.) The brain sciences are the fastest-developing area of medical science, and I believe that any doctor who prescribes antidepressants has an obligation to keep abreast of breaking events and research in this area.

In general, the doctor you will need to help guide you through the Antidepressant Survival Program should have an active and curious mind and be open to new ideas. He or she should be capable of unashamedly saying those three daunting words "I don't know"—but never "There is nothing that can be done." Whomever you select, he or she should be available by phone between visits to answer the brief questions that may arise as you proceed with the program.

RECRUITING YOUR DOCTOR TO MY PROGRAM

Your doctor may be a psychiatrist, an internist, a primary-care physician, or some sort of specialist, such as an endocrinologist. Any of these health professionals can work with you to maximize the benefits of the program—if they are open to learning from an outside source. This is a big *if.* In real life the mainstream sources of information most doctors review include a few journals, a few conferences, and perhaps a book in their area of interest. In psychiatry these mainstream sources of information are dominated by the pharmaceutical industry and, for lack of a better word, biological researchers.

Despite the overwhelming scientific evidence that the various systems of the body interact with one another constantly, there is a real scarcity of information from other fields in the mainstream information channels. This narrow, nonintegrative viewpoint—treating depression without knowledge of the entire chain of events leading up to it, which includes nutrition, hormones, immunology, and so on, as well as psychosocial-spiritual issues—limits the problem-solving ability of most doctors treating depression. Your doctor must be able to think "out of the box" to some degree; he or she must be aware that there may be other useful points of view, other valuable sources of knowledge.

Some doctors appreciate proactive patients who take the trouble to educate themselves about the medical underpinnings of their condition. Others, frankly, feel threatened by such patients. The advent of the Internet as a source of medical information for patients is a good case in point. Some doctors I speak to are delighted when their patients use the Web to educate themselves. Others express annoyance, along the lines of "Now every patient's an instant expert. They seem to forget that I'm the one who spent years training in my specialty."

The strength of my program lies in its integration of a wide range of medical specialties that affect, and are affected by, the action of your antidepressant medication: nutrition, exercise, psychopharmacology, endocrinology, immunology, and gastroenterology. It's likely that your doctor is *not* expert in one or more of these specialties. In order to endorse my program, your doctor needs to have confidence in the concepts, or needs to be curious enough to investigate for him- or herself, as I have done since 1979. Good doctors are always on the lookout for new treatment regimens that will benefit their patients. But they want to be assured that new therapies are based on good science.

I've taken care to address your doctor's concerns throughout this section of the book, citing sample studies that support a suggested treatment regimen as well as giving specific instructions on diagnosing and treating particular side effects. I've also written a special afterword to doctors, explaining my intent to supplement rather than replace their care and inviting them to contact me directly with follow-up questions or for professional training. Finally I have assembled an appendix with medical references that support the tenets of this program.

But despite the measures I've taken to anticipate your doctor's questions, you may encounter resistance when you approach your doctor with this book. Doctors, in common with all people, like to be valued. When you broach the Antidepressant Survival Program with your doctor, take care not to do so in a threatening or demanding fashion. Take pains to acknowledge each and every beneficial result your doctor's treatment has already afforded you. Elaborate on the positive aspects of your relationship with him or her. Do not allow your desire for a full life free from side effects to sound like an indictment of your doctor's compassion or skill.

Rather than arriving at your appointment and expecting your doctor to accept or reject this program on first sight, I suggest you send a copy of the book ahead and ask him or her to read through it in advance of your meeting. Or spend your first appointment explaining why you're interested in pursuing the program and plan to leave a copy for your doctor to read before your next meeting. Point out the most relevant medical sections, as well as the appendices and the address of my Website (www.wholepsych.com), where more diagnostic information and medical journal references are available.

Many people feel intimidated by their doctors; others are fearful of hurting their doctors' feelings. You might resent having to take your doctor's feelings into account. As with every other aspect of my program, pragmatism should be your prime directive when introducing your doctor to my program.

If facing your doctor directly is difficult, you should strongly consider the assistance of your therapist, pastor, sibling, or spouse. Discuss your concerns with your support person first, and consider how he or she might pave the way for you with your doctor. For example, your therapist could contact your doctor on your behalf by phone or (less desirably) by letter. She could explain your concerns and the serious impact they are having on your quality of life, and prepare your doctor for your visit, mentioning this book and your interest in getting your doctor's help in implementing this program. Your therapist can also serve a very useful purpose as a coach throughout this lifestyle change— if she understands the program and the problems you are facing.

To help you prepare for a successful first discussion with your doctor, I've created a sample script.

Dr. Jones: Hello, Nancy. What seems to be the problem today?

You: Dr. Jones, you know about the side effects I've been having from my medication. [If there are some you've never discussed before, this is the time.]

Dr. Jones: Yes. I see from your chart that you've gained some weight and report having less interest in sex...

You: I'm aware that our primary concern has been controlling my depression [or other symptoms for which you are taking the antidepressants]. And I'm tremendously relieved to have that nightmare behind me. I feel like the medication you've prescribed is my lifeline, and you have helped me immensely. I expect to stay on it for the foreseeable future, which is why I want to take the next step. I want to figure out how to minimize the side effects and maximize the benefits of the medicine.

Dr. Jones: All medications have side effects. There really isn't much we can do about them. I think you should keep them in perspective. Putting on a little weight and giving up some sexual pleasure is a small price to pay for curing depression. Unfortunately, our medical arsenal is limited.

You: It certainly feels like I'm making progress, but I want to take the next step toward a more fulfilling life. My loss of interest in sex is really taking its toll on my marriage. And it doesn't help that I feel overweight and unattractive.

Dr. Jones: I always advise my patients to keep to a healthy weight. Maybe you should try eating less or exercising more.

You: That's what I wanted to talk to you about. I read a book by a psychopharmacologist. He's developed a medical program that's specifically designed to enhance the benefits and minimize the side effects of antidepressants. Diet and exercise are part of his program, but there's also a medical component that includes testing for hormonal and dietary deficiencies.

Dr. Jones: Who is this doctor?

You: He's a professor of psychiatry at Georgetown University Hospital. He's also written a professional book about psychopharmacology called *Understanding Biological Psychiatry.* His program has worked for hundreds of his own patients on antidepressants. Since he encourages readers to enlist the active participation of their doctors, I wanted to talk to you about working with me on this program.

Dr. Jones: Well, I'd have to review his program before I could form an opinion.

You: I brought a copy of the book to leave with you. I'd appreciate it very much if you would read it. I've marked the special sections addressed to doctors. You'll see that he cites research studies his program is based on.

Dr. Jones (perusing the contents): This looks like a pretty ambitious plan.

You: I've read through it thoroughly, and it really speaks to my condition. I'm committed to trying it—but I need your help. I'd like to come back in a couple of weeks to discuss the program further, after you have had a chance to read it.

A conversation like this one makes it clear that you're asking your doctor's cooperation, not your doctor's permission. And it places the responsibility squarely on his shoulders to respond in a constructive way. This doesn't guarantee that your doctor will agree to help. But if he doesn't, you can feel confident that you've made your best effort to reach out and invite his participation.

If your doctor agrees to become your partner in undertaking the program, you're on your way. But what if he or she doesn't?

While I recognize that you may feel deeply invested in your current relationship with your doctor, you need to find a medical partner who takes your problems seriously and is committed to working with you toward a solution. If you hit a wall with your doctor, I suggest you ask for a referral to a doctor who will be more receptive. If that approach doesn't bear fruit, Appendix One will help you locate doctors who are sophisticated about psychopharmacology and receptive to this program.

In the meantime, despite the impasse you may have reached, you should feel free to maintain your relationship with your current doctor. For instance, if he's a psychiatrist with whom you have an ongoing and useful therapy schedule, you can continue seeing him while working with another doctor on my program. The important thing to keep in mind is that your doctor works for you. You are fully entitled to terminate the relationship whenever you like, *or accept the help he offers and go elsewhere for the additional help you need.* Just be sure that you don't terminate your relationship until you have a new doctor who can continue to prescribe your antidepressant medication.

In order to succeed at the Antidepressant Survival Program, you need a partnership with your doctor that is built on trust, communication, and mutual respect. You must believe in your doctor's caring, judgment, and skill, and your doctor must believe in your commitment to follow through with the program. Your doctor will also need to familiarize himself with the diagnostic tests and remedies prescribed in this program—many of which may be new to him—and will need to work with you closely, and on an ongoing basis, to achieve the best results. You have a right to that expectation. It is, lest you forget, why you are paying him.

Once you have a medical partner in your corner, you're ready to embark on the program. All you need is the resolve to get a life!

CHAPTER EIGHT

The Hormone Connection

* * *

THIS CHAPTER DEALS WITH hormone imbalances, the most common medical problem associated with antidepressant use. Imbalances often occur in the thyroid and adrenal systems, both of which are covered in this chapter. Imbalances in hormones related to appetite and blood sugar are described in the chapter that follows.

I have been astonished to find that at least 80 percent of my patients have abnormal functioning of the adrenal system and about 30 percent have disturbances in the thyroid system. The very fact that you're taking antidepressants places you in a high-risk category for some sort of hormone abnormality. Antidepressant use may be associated with an increased risk of thyroid dysfunction and impaired insulin or blood-sugar control—which in turn can affect your adrenal and thyroid glands.

Hormone imbalances can rob you of energy, sexual vitality, and feelings of well-being. They can also lead to weight gain and dull your thought processes. The bottom line is: hormonal problems can compound the side effects of antidepressants and can sabotage the beneficial effects of the Fundamentals. This is why I urge you to have your hormone systems tested. *There's no reason why you should continue to suffer from antidepressant side effects or incomplete response when there are simple, noninvasive ways to treat hormone imbalances.*

Consider Rhonda, who was a thirty-nine-year-old mother of two when she first came to see me three years ago. Rhonda had been taking

Zoloft, which her psychiatrist had prescribed for her depression six months earlier. Although she began to sleep better and didn't feel the same crushing sense of disappointment after a minor mishap at work, she found that she still wasn't able to shake the blues. She would force a smile as she tickled her two-year-old daughter and felt only apathy when thinking about an upcoming night out at her favorite restaurant. She told me that she just didn't enjoy pleasurable things the way she did before she got depressed. Rhonda had considered going off antidepressants when her doctor urged her to come to me. "Not only am I not being helped enough by the medication," she said, "but I'm actually feeling more tired than ever. I have trouble carrying a bag of groceries, and I feel like I'm moving in slow motion."

Based on her symptoms and my physical examination, I suspected that Rhonda's tiredness and lingering depression could be the results of an underactive thyroid system. So I took blood tests to measure her levels of thyroid hormones. My assumption proved correct, and I treated Rhonda with thyroid hormone pills and told her to continue taking the Zoloft. Within a few weeks she noticed a dramatic difference in her moods. She was once again able to anticipate and enjoy the time she spent with her family and friends.

HORMONE IMBALANCES

Hormones are major links in the mind-body connection. They are the chemical messengers that can turn on and off a variety of genes in every cell in your body. We also know that *all hormone imbalances may manifest as psychiatric disorders,* such as depression, mania, anxiety, attention deficit, memory disturbances, dementia, and even psychosis. *Hormone imbalances also mimic the side effects of antidepressants by causing weight gain, brain fog, sexual problems, and depleted energy levels.* Hormonal problems go hand in hand with depression, and sorting out "hormone-triggered" depression from clinical depression is not always easy. I usually find that my patients have a mixture of the two. For this reason, I strongly believe that a detailed assessment of the hormone systems should be a routine part of every psychiatric evaluation.

I often explain to my patients that neurotransmitters (for example, serotonin and norepinephrine) and hormones act as the body's shock absorber system. We all drive down the road of life, and we hit pot-holes. If our shock absorbers are functioning well, it's like we're driving a Cadillac. We feel the pothole, but only for a brief time, then we make a quick recovery. If we have poor shock absorbers, we feel like we're driving an old pickup truck. We hit the pothole, are stunned by it, and may veer off the road.

What determines how our shock absorbers work? Some of it is genetic, and some of it is set by the stress or trauma of very early life. In addition to nutritional and chemical factors, social environments play a significant role, as do our attitudes and interpretations of events.

Your body's glands take their cues from your brain, which deter-mines the exact timing and amount of hormones that should be released into your blood. By the same token, your brain gets a message from your glands (via your blood) providing a status update on hor-mone production and release. The relay of chemical signals between your brain and your glands keeps your body functioning properly. But this system's equilibrium can be upset when you take a blow from, say, depression or chronic pain or stress. In fact, hormonal imbalances are a major reason why antidepressants don't provide complete relief from depression or other medical conditions. So if you're depressed, your brain relays this message to your glands, which alter their production of hormones. On the flip side, if you have a malfunction in one of your glands, your brain will get a message and may respond by causing a partial shutdown in some of your systems, which can make you feel depressed.

Before we move into the heart of this chapter, let me comment on some of the latest research on our chemical environment and hormone disrupters. As you will note in other parts of this book, I am a strong advocate of organically grown (free from pesticides, fungicides, herbi-cides, and hormones) foods. Aside from the evidence suggesting organic foods' superior nutritional content, and the definite health ben-efits seen in experimental animals, there is growing concern that the chemicals we accept in our environment are a significant cause of hor-monal problems in the population at large, by mimicking or blocking the functions of our own hormone systems. I have often wondered if the frequency of hormonal problems in the people I work with is related to the chemical environment, and if that is not in some way also responsible for the steady rise in the incidence of depression over the last several decades. I do not know the answer for sure, but I for one prefer not to wait the ten or twenty years it may take to find out. That's why I strongly suggest that you eat organic foods whenever possible.

This chapter is divided into two parts: thyroid and adrenal system abnormalities. The chapter that follows will deal with blood-sugar abnormalities. At the beginning of each part, take the self-evaluation quiz to see if you are experiencing symptoms that need to be further evaluated by your doctor.

YOUR THYROID HORMONES
Hypothyroidism

An underactive thyroid, also called hypothyroidism, can be caused by antidepressants. Although researchers don't understand how antidepressants suppress thyroid function, they've known for years that lithium can cause hypothyroidism and have recently implicated other antidepressants as well. Hypothyroidism can also occur on its own— because of diet (for instance, inadequate minerals, vitamins, essential fatty acids, amino acids, or excess carbohydrates), an immune reaction, genetic susceptibility, or from radiation treatments for an overactive thyroid.

Regardless of the cause, hypothyroidism can lead to numerous problems, including but not limited to weight gain, excessive tiredness, decreased sexual function, and brain fog—all of which can mimic antidepressant side effects. The condition can also *cause* depressed moods and render antidepressants *ineffective.* So you may think your medication isn't working when the problem is actually caused by an inadequate level of thyroid hormones.

Many people on antidepressants who have symptoms of hypothyroidism may not have the full-blown condition that can be diagnosed using a standard blood test, which measures the level of thyroid-stimulating hormone (TSH). Instead, they have a milder form of the condition called subclinical hypothyroidism. In the late 1980s I became frustrated after the test results of many of my patients with multiple symptoms of hypothyroidism kept coming back normal. This can't be right, I thought. I decided to perform a thyroid-releasing hormone

(TRH) stimulation test, a much more sensitive test that can detect subtle abnormalities in one part of the thyroid system—the pituitary gland's responsiveness to the hypothalamus.

I hired an independent statistician to review the records of one hundred patients who initially had normal results based on the standard thyroid test, but who underwent additional thyroid testing, including the TRH stimulation test. I was astounded when the statistician called me with the results. *Fifty percent of the patients I tested turned out to have subclinical hypothyroidism!* The findings were also confirmed clinically, after my patients noticed a clear improvement in their mental sluggishness, weight, and energy levels, as well as numerous other symptoms (one patient's periodontal surgery was canceled when her gums were restored to normal) after they were treated with thyroid hormone. What concerns me most is that *doctors who rely on the results of the routine blood test are missing many cases of hypothyroidism in patients on antidepressants.*

The classic signs of hypothyroidism include sluggishness, muscle fatigue, cold sensitivity, constipation, irregular menstrual periods, dry skin, mental fuzziness, and weight gain—which can be upwards of twenty pounds. These symptoms are vague and can be indicative of a host of other medical conditions. For this reason, about half of the 11 million Americans who have hypothyroidism go undiagnosed because they mistakenly attribute their symptoms to normal aging, stress, or menopause. I'd estimate that missed diagnoses are even more common in people who take antidepressants, since their doctors may attribute their hypothyroid symptoms to antidepressant side effects.

Unfortunately, many doctors still aren't aware of the connection between antidepressant use and hypothyroidism. If you are experiencing thyroid symptoms, you may need to be persistent to get your doctor to order the appropriate tests. If your request for testing is denied, make sure your doctor supplies a reason beyond "It isn't necessary." If you're not satisfied with your doctor's answer, find a doctor who will give you the tests you need.

GETTING TESTED FOR HYPOTHYROIDISM

If you answer yes to two or more questions in the thyroid quiz that follows, I recommend a blood test to measure levels of three hormones:

Thyroid Self-Evaluation

1. Do you feel like you have weak muscles (especially in your upper arms and thighs) when you do simple physical tasks like climbing stairs, getting up from a chair, or styling your hair?

2. Have you recently had an unexplained weight gain, despite eating the same amount or even a little less than usual?

3. Do you always feel cold? (For instance, you need to wear a sweater when others do not, or you keep your thermostat set higher than seventy-two degrees.)

4. Do your nails break easily?

5. Is your skin dry?

6. Do you notice that you're shedding more hair than usual?

7. Are you often constipated?

8. Do you have swelling in your hands or feet or puffiness below your eyes?

9. Do you have irregular menstrual periods or infertility problems?

10. Is your antidepressant medication only partly effective?

If you answer Yes to two or more of these questions, you need to find out if you have an underactive thyroid. Read the section on hypothyroidism.

thyroid-stimulating hormone (TSH), free thyroxine (T_4), and free tri-iodothyronine (T_3). As I explained in the previous section the standard test, which measures just TSH, is not always sufficient, since TSH levels can be normal even when the thyroid is underactive. This is why I strongly recommend that your doctor perform the more comprehensive testing that measures all three hormones. (I have more on this in Note to Your Doctor on page 180.)

Four days before you see your doctor to have your blood drawn, you need to begin taking your temperature three times a day. Make a written record of your temperatures (include the dates and times), and give this record to your doctor. Take your oral temperature with a standard or digital mercury thermometer, and record the reading to one-tenth of a degree. Take the first reading three hours after waking, the second three hours later, and the third three hours later. If you wake up at, say, 7:00 A.M., you would take your temperature at 10:00 A.M., 1:00 P.M., and 4:00 P.M.

The purpose of these temperature recordings is to determine the overall effectiveness of your thyroid system in controlling your metabolism. Since most of us—with the exception of some lawyers—are warm-blooded creatures, our bodies function best in a narrow temperature range. (When we get a fever of even half a degree above normal, we may feel a change in our sense of well-being.)

If you have an overactive thyroid system, it will increase your body's metabolism, raising your temperature significantly above the normal 98.6 degrees. If too little hormone is available, your metabolism will decrease, causing your temperature to drop below normal.

Note: Your temperature can be affected by various factors, such as having a cold, being premenstrual, exercising, or eating hot or cold foods fifteen to thirty minutes before taking your temperature. Try to record your temperature before mealtimes and exercise, and (if you're a woman) during the first half of your cycle.

NOTE TO YOUR DOCTOR

Adequate Assessment of the Thyroid Axis

Studying the physiology of the thyroid axis makes it clear that a simple TSH level—even the most sophisticated kind—is not a fully adequate test of the thyroid system, unless one is screening for only advanced cases of thyroid dysfunction. As an example, if you suspect subclinical hypothyroidism, a well-established phenomenon, a TSH is not sufficient because it indicates only the output of the pituitary gland. In cases when the pituitary or hypothalamus is suboptimally responsive to a low-normal free T_4 or free T_3, then the TSH can be normal or high normal and the patient can still be subclinically hypothyroid. Thus I recommend that every patient with signs and/or symptoms of hypothyroidism be tested with body temperatures (see the preceding section) as well as TSH, free T_4, and free T_3 (use the free tests to eliminate protein-binding distortions of test results). These results need to be looked at along with baseline temperature recordings and physical examination.

A patient with suggestive signs (including palpation for nodules and goiter) or symptoms may have subclinical hypothyroidism if any of the three hormones mentioned are near the limits of normal, if they are abnormal, or if temperature recordings are consistently averaging about one degree below normal. In addition, after observing thyroid hormone lab results for several years, I have come to see that the relationship of the hormones to one another must also be taken into account. For example, a consistently low-normal free T_4 with a low-normal TSH indicates either a low set point or a relative failure of positive feedback to the pituitary and/or hypothalamus. A midrange to high-normal free T_4 and a low-normal TSH may indicate a tendency to an overactive gland, which the hypothalamic-pituitary portions of the system are compensating for. A free T_4 and TSH in the fiftieth percentile of normal in the presence of a free T_3 in the tenth percentile of normal indicates the possibility of a relatively poor conversion of T_4 to T_3 in the periphery. In this case, even though all the more central parts of the thyroid axis are intact, some peripheral disturbance in conversion may be accounting for your patient's sluggishness, failure to respond to antidepressants, presumed side effects of the medication, and so on.

If test results indicate hypothyroidism, it is standard to test for thyroid peroxidase or antimicrosomal antibodies to rule out Hashimoto's thyroiditis. In addition, the patient should be tested for an adrenal axis abnormality and have a thyroid scan if enlargement or thyroid nodule is suspected (see my recommendations for adrenal testing on page 186). Adrenal axis malfunctions often go hand in hand with hypothyroidism. For instance, increased cortisol is associated with a lower body temperature set point and lower levels of free T_3, two of the indicators used in assessing thyroid function (L. Bartalena, et al., *Journal of Clinical Endocrinology and Metabolism* 70, 1990: 293).

Subclinical hypothyroidism (low to low-normal levels of free T_3 or T_4) is common in patients exhibiting depressive symptoms or other symptoms of hypothyroidism and requires treatment even if TSH levels are within the normal range. One study found that 56 percent of people with subclinical hypothyroidism suffered from depression compared with a rate of 20 percent in the average population (J. J. Haggerth, et al., *American Journal of Psychiatry* 150, no. 3, March 1993: 508–10). Many of these patients go on to develop full-blown hypothyroidism.

If your patient has signs of subclinical hypothyroidism (thyroid signs and symptoms, normal TSH, low-range free T_3 or low-range free T_4, and perhaps basal body temperature one degree below normal on average), I recommend referring the patient to an endocrinologist to perform a thyroid-releasing hormone (TRH) stimulation test to assess the pituitary and hypothalamic aspects of thyroid axis function.

One study found that 19 percent of patients who had subclinical hypothyroidism diagnosed using a TRH stimulation test had had an episode of major depression within the past year, compared with none of the subjects with a normal TRH stimulation test (J. J. Haggerth, et al., above). Nearly all of my symptomatic patients who have a normal TSH and low-normal free T_4 and free T_3 but an abnormal result on the TRH stimulation test had clinically significant improvement in their sluggishness, weight, depressed moods, and other signs and symptoms after being treated with synthetic thyroid hormone.

TREATMENT FOR HYPOTHYROIDISM

If you are diagnosed with an underactive thyroid, your doctor will probably prescribe levothyroxine (Synthroid or Levoxyl), a synthetic version of T_4 or thyroxine. Synthroid is one of the five most commonly prescribed medications in the United States. Other medications, such as triiodothyronine (Cytomel), contain just T_3. Your doctor can also prescribe T_4 and T_3 pills in combination. I will explain the pros and cons of the various treatment options in the following Note to Your Doctor. Realize that your doctor may feel it is best if your treatment is managed by an endocrinologist. If this happens, I strongly advise you to find someone who specializes in thyroid problems and is aware of the overlap with psychiatric illness and medication efficacy.

Beyond medicinal treatments, you should be vigilant about following the Fundamentals, especially the nutrition and exercise components. Having a diet that's too high in carbohydrates or depleted of certain micronutrients can reduce your body's ability to manufacture T_4 or T_3. Exercise can improve your energy levels and help you maintain a healthy weight.

NOTE TO YOUR DOCTOR

Treatment for Hypothyroidism

Once you have ascertained that your patient has hypothyroidism and have assessed the possible causes, you must decide the best course of treatment—and this is not always easy. Your patient can be treated with T_4 (levothyroxine) or T_3 (triiodothyronine) or a combination. There is good clinical evidence that using a combination of T_3 and T_4 can help alleviate symptoms of depression in patients with hypothyroidism who have had only a partial response to antidepressants (*Journal of Clinical*

Psychiatry 53, no. 1, January 1992: 16–18) and improve neurocognitive function. ("Effects of thyroxine as compared with thyroxine plus triiodothyronine in patients with hypothyroidism," *New England Journal of Medicine* 340, no. 6, February 11, 1999: 424–29).

If you elect to begin the standard treatment of levothyroxine, you should periodically take blood samples to monitor levels of free T_4, free T_3, and TSH; the TSH level should not drop below .05 because of the increased risk of osteoporosis and, of course, the possibility of inducing iatrogenic hyperthyroidism.

With time you may note that the thyroid symptoms or the depression recur, which means you'll need to recheck the thyroid axis and possibly raise the dosage of levothyroxine. In these situations I advise you to monitor your patient's body temperature (as discussed on page 179) and check levels of TSH, free T_4, and free T_3 again. If the levels of T_3 are low to low-normal, while TSH and free T_4 are clearly normal, you should start supplementing with T_3. Despite the fact that Cytomel is reported to have a long half-life, requiring only once-daily dosing, I have found that trough blood levels of free T_3 are often low within twelve hours of taking the Cytomel, even with twice-daily dosing. For this reason, when finances allow, I use a form of T_3 compounded in a slow-release base by a compounding pharmacy. This is taken every twelve hours in 7.5-microgram increments, and dosage is determined by following the body temperature as well as the peak (six hours after dose) and trough (twelve hours after dose) free T_3. As always, one must be sure that the TSH is not overly suppressed to avoid increased risk of osteoporosis. This approach seems to keep the blood levels of T_3 more constant and frequently improves sleep, energy, other symptoms, and response to the antidepressant. Researchers have also found thyroid intervention helpful in managing attention deficit disorder associated with depression. This is not surprising given the essential role of T_3 in catecholamine signaling pathways.

Adrenal Self-Evaluation

1. Do you crave salty foods?

2. Do you feel so tired that you have difficulty making it through the day?

3. Do you feel dizzy or light-headed when you stand up?

4. Do you feel muscle fatigue when performing everyday tasks?

5. Do you have difficulty concentrating?

6. Have you experienced an unexplained weight gain, particularly in your face, midsection, and back of your neck?

7. Do you have appetite loss, difficulty gaining weight, or frequent nausea?

8. Have you noticed any of the following changes in skin coloration: age spots; dark lines in or around your nails; darkening of the skin around your elbows, knuckles, knees, or nipples; a tan that doesn't fade normally; darkening of the creases on your palms; or purple streaks on your abdomen?

9. Have your periods become less frequent or disappeared entirely?

10. Do you bruise easily, heal slowly, or notice thinning of your skin?

11. Do you get any of the following symptoms—irritability, shakiness, dizziness, nausea, light-headedness, sweatiness, headache—if you miss a meal or go more than three hours without eating *and* do you find that these symptoms are alleviated by food?

If you answered yes to two or more questions, you may have an adrenal system abnormality. Read the accompanying section on adrenal disorders. If you answered yes to question 11, you may also have hypoglycemia. This condition is covered in Chapter 9.

ADRENAL GLANDS:
HOW ARE YOUR SHOCK ABSORBERS?

There are numerous types of adrenal system abnormalities. Since certain kinds of adrenal system abnormalities frequently go hand in hand with thyroid problems, I routinely test patients with hypothyroidism for adrenal gland problems and vice versa. Adrenal problems are very common during an episode of depression. They often linger, however, even after treatment with antidepressants. As I mentioned earlier, I've found that at least 80 percent of my patients have abnormal levels (high and low) and abnormal rhythms of adrenal hormones. Such abnormalities are associated with weight gain and blood-sugar and insulin disturbances, sleep disruptions, low energy levels, immune dysfunction, and reduced sex drive—all of which can exacerbate the side effects and minimize the benefits of antidepressants.

Why is the adrenal system taking such a hit? Your adrenal glands are designed to help you react to an acute stress, like a sudden interpersonal conflict or a car cutting in front of you on the highway. In this type of situation, they pump out the hormone adrenaline, which quickens your heartbeat and pulse, accelerates your breathing rate, and instantaneously reroutes your blood to prepare your muscles and brain for quick action.

In addition to helping you deal with acute stress, your adrenal glands respond more gradually to long-term and repeated stresses, such as depression, chronic pain, or illness. In this situation the glands begin to pump out abnormally high amounts of another hormone, cortisol. This hormone is normally released in larger amounts in the morning and steadily decreasing amounts through the day, until it is at its low point at 4:00 A.M. With depression and, often, chronic illness, however, cortisol release is out of rhythm. It may be too low in the morning (which leaves you feeling drowsy) and too high in the evening (which can make you feel too alert at bedtime). Basically, you feel jet-lagged because your body's internal clock has gone off its normal daily cycle. You may have trouble sleeping, feel fatigued, and have difficulty concentrating.

Another common adrenal system abnormality is high levels of cortisol throughout the day and night. This pattern can cause you to gain fat while losing muscle, which is one way adrenal gland problems can lead to weight gain. With chronic, prolonged stress, your body produces too much cortisol. *Excess cortisol can harm some of the cells involved in memory storage* as well as cause a multitude of other problems, such as ulcers, osteoporosis, and weight gain. The increase in cortisol is counterbalanced by a reduction in the adrenal output of DHEA, a precursor to the sex hormones. As a result you may have a diminished sex drive and another cause of weight gain and muscle loss. (You may also have reduced immune function.) It's as if your adrenals are saying: "It's time to worry about survival—let's put sex on the back burner."

If stress and poor nutrition continue long enough, the output of cortisol will eventually drop below normal—as will DHEA and other adrenal hormones—putting you into a state called adrenal fatigue (a severe form of which is called Addison's disease).

By normalizing your body's reaction to stress, antidepressants can help shift your adrenal gland function back to normal—but often not completely.

GETTING TESTED FOR ADRENAL PROBLEMS

The easiest, most information-packed, and most reliable screening test for assessing how your adrenal system and glands are functioning is called an adrenal stress index (ASI). This test measures the amount of two hormones: free cortisol (which means it is unbound and able to be taken up by the brain) and DHEA. The ASI requires you to donate a little saliva (into a tube) at four specified times over the course of a day.

It measures the rises and dips of cortisol and DHEA through the day, so that both hormonal rhythm and level can be gauged.

The ASI is more specific than the standard adrenal test, which your doctor may want to perform—a twenty-four-hour urinary free cortisol test. This test requires you to collect all your urine over the course of a day (which is a much bigger hassle than simply spitting into a tube), and it measures only the total amount of free cortisol. The test can't measure the actual rise and decline of cortisol through the day, so rhythm abnormalities cannot be assessed. Some people may have a normal test result even though their adrenal glands may be releasing too much cortisol at night and not enough in the morning. If your doctor has difficulty finding a laboratory that runs the ASI test, I provide the name and address of the laboratory I use in Appendix One.

NOTE TO YOUR DOCTOR

Benefits of the Adrenal Stress Index

When I first considered using the ASI in my clinical practice, I was discouraged by a few endocrinologists, whose impressions were that the test was essentially worthless. One very competent endocrinologist quoted Robert Post, M.D., of the National Institutes of Health, and pointed out that the test was abandoned by NIH because of its uselessness. I performed a thorough literature search, because I didn't want to discard such a potentially information-packed and easy test. As it turned out, not only was there a great deal of substantive, high-quality research supporting the validity and reliability of this test but a significant contribution to this literature was made by Dr. Post (J. P. Kahn, D. R. Rubinow, C. L. Davis, M. Kling, and R. Post, "Salivary cortisol: A practical method for evaluation of adrenal function," *Biological Psychiatry* 23, 1988: 335–49). Confused by the conflict between the research and the clinical endocrinologists' attitudes, I called Dr. Post. He confirmed my understanding of the literature and explained that NIH had abandoned the test because their patient population was actually living at the institute. For a variety of reasons, it was easier for them to do blood testing at any hour of the day or night that they chose. Finally, to check the accuracy and reliability of the laboratory I use, I have sent multiple duplicate samples, submitted under different names, as I do with all the laboratories I use. (I abandon those laboratories that come up with inaccurate results.)

It is clear that the salivary levels of cortisol, DHEA, and sex hormones correlate well with the blood levels of the free bioactive hormone concentration. It is the free fraction that we are concerned with for a number of reasons, including the fact that only the free form is taken up by the brain, where these hormones are biologically active.

Serum cortisol levels reflect only total concentrations, including protein-bound portions, at the moment of the blood drawing and do not give any information about diurnal variation in cortisol secretion patterns. Corticosteroids measured in twenty-four-hour urine collections obscure aberrant fluctuations in cortisol secretion at different times of the day.

The home saliva testing kit (ASI) affords the opportunity to obtain accurate, reliable, and patient-friendly real-life information on the adrenal axis that is not routinely available via other tests. The patterns of disruption of cortisol output as well as the magnitude of disruption offer very useful clinical information. Patterns of abnormal secretions can indicate sympathetic overdrive, hypoglycemia, and so on. For instance, when cortisol output is high at the 11:00 P.M. sample time, REM sleep is often diminished and sleep is unrefreshing. This pattern may be associated with an incompletely treated depression or be an early sign of relapse.

Additional information on the ASI includes the presence of antigliadin antibodies, high levels of which are correlated with fatigue (J. A. Arnason, *GUT* 33, no. 2, 1992: 194–97), and marginal or low B_{12}, folate, and ferritin status.

TREATING ADRENAL GLAND PROBLEMS

One of the benefits of the Fundamentals is that they help *gradually* reverse adrenal system malfunctions. *The nutrition plan* is designed to stabilize blood-sugar levels by limiting your intake of sugar, refined flour, and caffeine, all of which cause spikes in blood sugar, followed by quick plunges. These plunges trigger the release of adrenaline, which works to get more sugar into your bloodstream. By the same token, large amounts of sugar or starchy foods trigger your adrenal glands to release cortisol (stimulated by the release of insulin), which helps store the excess glucose as fat. This, of course, leads to weight gain around your midsection. The nutrition plan will help you avoid these sugar crashes by enabling you to eat balanced amounts of carbohydrates, protein, and fat, and help normalize your insulin and cortisol. (And, as I mentioned earlier, eating organic foods helps limit your exposure to hormone disrupters, which, in the susceptible individual, are suspected contributors to hormonal and psychiatric problems.)

The exercise program helps regulate your adrenal functioning by reducing the output of the stress hormones adrenaline and cortisol. It also helps reduce your appetite and can help you shed excess weight.

The relaxation-play-spirituality component of the Fundamentals has been proven to help the adrenal system recover by reducing stress. One interesting study from the University of Iowa found that doing Transcendental Meditation twice a day for fifteen to twenty minutes can help reverse the effects of chronic stress by lowering your adrenal glands' production of cortisol and other stress hormones. (See Chapter 6 for instructions on how to meditate.) I strongly recommend Transcendental Meditation (taught by a teacher) to my patients with adrenal dysfunction.

Vitamin and Mineral Supplements

Beyond following the Antidepressant Survival Program, I recommend taking the following vitamin and mineral supplements if you have an adrenal system abnormality. They are useful regardless of whether your adrenal system is overactive, underactive, or both. Stay on these supplements for six months to one year, or until you have your hormone levels retested—unless you have an adverse reaction. Add the supplements to your daily regimen one at a time, every three days, to detect any intolerances:

Pantothenic acid—500 milligrams, twice a day, with breakfast and dinner

Folic acid—800 micrograms, twice a day, with breakfast and dinner

B-Complex "50" (Solgar)—one capsule a day with a meal

Ester-C with bioflavonoids—1000 milligrams, twice a day with a meal

Zinc—25 milligrams, once a day on an empty stomach—preferably one to two hours after dinner or at bedtime

What to do if your cortisol levels are low: Low blood pressure (a reading below 110 over 70, which shows a drop of 10 points on standing) is one of the most problematic conditions associated with low adrenal output and causes dizziness on standing, fatigue, lightheadedness, and brain fog. The treatment is fairly simple: Increase the amount of salt in your diet. You can also take a 500-milligram salt tablet three to six times per day. If you decide to take these tablets, be sure to drink at least one full eight-ounce glass of water with every dose. If you can't get your blood pressure up with salt tablets, you can use licorice root extract, but beware that it can cause increased blood pressure and fluid retention. Licorice root extract should not be used during pregnancy, in the presence of liver disorders or low potassium levels, or by those on diuretics or digitalis. The benefits—and side effects—of licorice extract come on gradually and go away gradually. *This is a potent intervention that should be undertaken only with your doctor's supervision and approval.* As an alternative, your doctor may prescribe Flurinef, a medication that can help raise blood pressure after doing an ACTH stimulation test to determine the status of your adrenal gland itself.

Some doctors believe that hydrocortisone may help raise cortisol levels and alleviate the symptoms of reduced adrenal output. But the jury is still out on whether this treatment is actually beneficial. Moreover, hydrocortisone can cause a host of side effects, including stomach upset, high blood pressure, insomnia, weight gain, and muscle weakness—to name just a few. A recent study in *The New England Journal of Medicine* indicated hydrocortisone was ineffective, by objective measurement, in patients who had low adrenal function associated with chronic fatigue syndrome, although the study did find that some patients felt better after taking the hydrocortisone. This treatment is still controversial, but it may warrant a discussion with your doctor.

What to do if your cortisol levels are high: Your doctor needs to investigate why your cortisol levels are high or consider referring you to an endocrinologist or other specialist for further testing. You may have unresolved depression or hypoglycemia, or be under severe emotional stress. Or you may be experiencing chronic inflammation or pain. Your doctor also needs to rule out more serious medical conditions, such as Cushing's disease or congenital adrenal hyperplasia.

If your doctor concludes that your high cortisol levels are the result of your previous anxiety, depression, blood-sugar instabilities, chronic stress or pain, or other conditions, you should take a nutrient supplement called phosphatidyl serine (PS). This is a phospholipid that helps your brain cells respond normally to signals from the adrenal glands. Essentially, PS will help normalize your brain's responsiveness to adrenal hormones, so that if your levels of cortisol are high your brain won't send out a signal to your adrenals to produce more. If this doesn't work, DHEA or ketoconazole (Nizoral) may be considered.

The timing and amount of PS you should take depends on the time of day your cortisol levels peak and the number of peaks you have during the day. The lab that performs your ASI test will provide your doctor with a graph that shows your peaks. Take a 100-milligram dose of the supplement two hours before each of your cortisol peaks. You may need to take up to four doses per day, depending on how many peaks you have. About 10 minutes after taking a dose, make sure to eat a snack that contains at least one or two grams of fat; this will aid with the absorption of the supplement. For example, if you have a cortisol peak at 4:00 P.M. and one at midnight, you should take your PS at 2:00 P.M. and 10:00 P.M. Have a snack that contains some protein, carbohydrates, and fat at about 2:10 P.M. and 10:10 P.M. Some suggestions: a handful of mixed nuts and raisins, peanut butter on a rice cake, a one-ounce slice of cheese with three crackers.

Treatment for Adrenal Gland Problems

If your patient's adrenal profile is normal, with the exception of high levels of cortisol (escape) in the midnight sample, your patient probably has unresolved depression, which is often associated with REM sleep abnormalities. In the classic studies on endogenous depression, failure to suppress cortisol output was consistently found to be a strong predictor of relapse into depression. It is essential to normalize cortisol escape through changes in diet, lifestyle, and supplementation—or possibly a change in medication.

I recommend supplementation with phosphatidyl serine (PS), also referred to as phosphorylated serine. This supplement has been reported to help normalize feedback of the hypothalamic-pituitary-adrenal axis (D. Kretz, "Corticotropin-releasing hormone expression is the major target for glucocorticoid feedback-control at the hypothalamic level," *Brain Research* 818, no. 2, February 13, 1999: 488–91), enhance enzymes involved in monitoring neurotransmitter production and release, help neuronal glucose utilization, and modulate the fluidity of neuronal cell membranes. My patients have reported improved sleep and mood with this agent, and it seems to help reduce elevated cortisol levels.

Phosphatidyl serine should be given orally two hours before the steroid elevation, with a small amount of a high-fat food (such as nuts) ten minutes later to aid in the absorption. It can be used anytime throughout the day to bring down elevated cortisol levels. In addition to the fact that elevated cortisol levels are indicative of chronic stress, such levels are of concern because they place the patient at risk for increased damage to the hippocampal cells (which mediate memory) as well as other diseases.

If the cortisol is elevated throughout the day, PS may be given several times per day, about two hours before each cortisol peak.

The cause of the elevated steroid levels (e.g., depression, tumor, Cushing's disease, congenital adrenal hyperplasia, overexertion, medication, inflammation, hypoglycemia) should also be investigated. Finally, there is some preliminary evidence that treatment with DHEA or ketoconazole may reduce cortisol and alleviate depression.

If DHEA levels are low, supplementation with DHEA (15 to 50 milligrams taken at breakfast) is generally indicated in males. Use appropriate testing for prostate cancer, as well as follow-up ASI testing. In addition, once the patient is stabilized on a dose, a twenty-four-hour urine test for fractionated 17-ketosteroids should be obtained to ascertain that downstream metabolites of DHEA (such as etiocholanolone or androstenedione) are not elevated.

Women should not be placed on DHEA without a DHEA challenge test, which helps to determine the conversion pathways in the individual (how much DHEA is converted to estrogen and testosterone) and avoid potentially irreversible virilization. This test can be done, using a DHEA challenge test (DCT) kit, simply by taking a baseline level of salivary testosterone, estrogen, and DHEA. After five to seven days of supplementation with the planned DHEA dose, the tests should be repeated. Significant increases in testosterone or estrogen outside the normal ranges preclude the use of DHEA in some women. You may have greater success using sublingual forms of DHEA in women, with less conversion to estrogen and testosterone. Dosages of DHEA for women are in the 5- to 15-milligram range.

It is important to note that correction of diet alone through the Fundamentals nutrition plan outlined in Chapter 4 can double DHEA levels over three months, so if a doubling of the DHEA would put the patient in a sufficiently normal range, then dietary intervention alone could be a reasonable plan.

If the patient has orthostatic hypotension, which has been reported to be associated with chronic fatigue syndrome, consider using salt tablets, 500 to 1000 milligrams three times a day, licorice root extract (dried roots of *Glycyrrhiza glabra* containing glycyrrhizic acid) to stimulate mineralocorticoid production (200 to 600 milligrams of glycyrrhizin in the morning), or Flurinef (0.1 milligram per day).

Note: Licorice extract can cause edema and hypertension, hypokalemia, and, rarely, myoglobinuria. It should not be used in patients on potassium-depleting drugs (for example, thiazide diuretics) and may increase sensitivity to digitalis.

CHAPTER NINE

Gut
Reactions

* * *

YOUR DIGESTIVE SYSTEM is the foundation of your physical and emotional health. If your gastrointestinal system—defined as the "tube" (and its attachments, such as the pancreas and liver) that runs from the mouth to the anus—is failing you in some way, it will undermine your well-being on a number of levels.

Various problems can occur as your gut attempts to break down and absorb the foods you eat. Even one glitch in the system can begin a cascade that prevents nutrients from getting to your brain and other organs. Your body will slowly veer out of balance, and you'll eventually suffer from more than just indigestion. You may find that you have extreme side effects from antidepressants, because when your liver is short on essential nutrients it can't break down the medicines efficiently. Or your depression may linger on at a low level because some essential nutrients are in short supply, causing less than adequate nerve cell function. Or you may develop low energy levels and a significant midafternoon energy slump. As surprising as it may seem, your digestive health is vital for having a balanced body and for living a full life.

In Chapter 4 I talked about how you are what you eat and how giving your body the proper fuel will help balance your body's systems. Let me clarify this a little: You are what you eat—but only to the degree that your cells receive the nutrients from your food. Sometimes the gut can't digest food well enough to deliver on this basic requirement of health. So even if you're following the eating plan outlined in the Fundamentals, you may not be able to restore balance to your body and mind without also helping your gastrointestinal tract to do its job well. This is a fairly common problem: *I would estimate that 25 percent of my patients have some disturbance in their digestive systems that causes symptoms and reduces their ability to properly utilize the foods they eat.*

Let me explain a bit about how your digestive system works. The gastrointestinal tract is essentially a twenty-five- to thirty-foot-long tube that passes food from one end of your body to the other. In a sense, your gastrointestinal tract is like the hole in a donut, actually distinct from the donut (your body). The gastrointestinal tract is an independent entity, with a great deal of its activity dictated by its own semi-independent nervous system.

In a simplistic sense, the tube is lined with what I will call gatekeeper cells and secretory cells. The gatekeeper cells determine what is allowed into your bloodstream. These cells are pretty picky. They keep indigestible foreign substances (like insoluble fiber found in vegetables and fruits or large proteins) from entering the bloodstream. Gatekeeper cells receive much nourishment from the contents of the gastrointestinal tract, including the friendly bacteria that help digest the food as it gets squeezed down the tube by the rhythmic churning of your digestive muscles.

As the food is being broken down into smaller parts, the secretory cells (there are many types) squirt out protective mucus, as well as digestive enzymes and juices to break these parts down further into nutrients and vitamins, which are then allowed to pass through to your bloodstream.

Once the food has passed through this first checkpoint, it faces another round of inspection by your immune cells. *This line of defense is so important that 50 to 60 percent of our immune system actually surrounds the gastrointestinal tract.* These immune cells label as invaders any unwanted bacteria, viruses, and parasites, as well as partially digested proteins that somehow made it through the first checkpoint. The immune cells can't send these unwanted invaders back to where they came from, so they mount an attack instead. The white blood cells are called into action to neutralize these enemies.

Depending on the intensity of the immune system's reaction, you may experience anything from mild sluggishness and brain fog (from the release of chemicals called cytokines, which can affect how your brain functions) to an intense, classic allergic reaction. Tissues anywhere in your body may become inflamed or achy. When your digestive system (gatekeeper cells, secretory cells, muscles, and associated glands and organs) and immune cells work as they should, the right nutrients get to the cells in your body.

When one part of this assembly line is malfunctioning, however, the whole digestion and absorption process, as well as brain function and sense of well-being, can be affected. As an example, if the secretory cells in your stomach are not releasing enough acid (maybe you take a lot of Tums or an antacid medication, or perhaps there is some other problem), then the stomach enzyme (pepsinogen) cannot be changed into its active form (pepsin), which is necessary to start the breaking down of protein and the release of other downstream digestive enzymes.

DIGESTION AND ANTIDEPRESSANTS

Why is healthy digestive function so important to people on antidepressants? Because without the breakdown of protein into peptides, and then into even smaller amino acids, your brain cells will not get one of the most important building blocks of the brain chemical serotonin. When protein is broken down into its building block amino acids, it creates tryptophan (one of the so-called essential amino acids you can get only from food). Tryptophan then enters the blood and travels to the brain cells, where it is made into serotonin. If you don't have enough tryptophan, you can't make enough serotonin, and you can become depressed.

At that point, let's assume you go to your doctor, who prescribes an SSRI, like Prozac or Luvox. The medication cannot and will not work, since there is not enough serotonin being manufactured by your brain. In a similar manner, if your gastrointestinal tract is failing to break down and absorb other foods, vitamins, and minerals, then nutrients vital to your mind-body functions will also not be absorbed into your bloodstream.

Patients with nutritional deficiencies are frequently told they have "treatment-resistant" depression. *At least 70 percent of the patients who come to me with treatment-resistant depression actually have some type of nutrient deficiency—such as low levels of essential fatty acids or zinc—that is at least partly responsible for their inadequate response to medication.*

Finally, even if the proper nutrients actually get into your bloodstream, your body may not be able to deal with certain foods. For instance, eating an excessive amount of sweets can, in some people, cause an insulin reaction and hypoglycemia, a condition in which the body fails to maintain a steady blood-sugar level. Recently evidence has emerged that confirms what many of my patients already know: Some psychotropic medications can alter blood-sugar regulation. Clinical evidence suggests that further research will indicate this problem may be caused by some antidepressants as well.

EVALUATING YOUR GUT REACTIONS: THREE BASIC TESTS

This chapter will tell you how to assess and treat
  1. Digestive abnormalities
  2. Hypoglycemia
  3. Food allergies and sensitivities

I've included a self-evaluation quiz at the beginning of each section to help you identify which, if any, of these problems you have. I then detail the specific diagnostic tests and treatments you need.

Regardless of your symptoms, though, I strongly recommend that you have the following three blood tests. Even in the absence of gastrointestinal tract symptoms, they will shed light on your nutritional and, to a lesser degree, immune system status. These tests can give your doctor information on your particular condition and can also uncover hidden conditions that may be masquerading as depression or as antidepressant side effects.

I feel these three tests are so important that I give them to all my patients—even those who aren't experiencing symptoms of gastrointestinal problems. I'm frequently dismayed to see nutritional deficiencies in patients who are eating what appear to be fairly well-balanced diets. This is why I'm convinced that it's not enough simply to tell your doctor what you're eating. You and your doctor need to find out how your body is digesting the foods you eat.

Some of these tests are fairly standard and are performed by most laboratories throughout the country. For the specialty tests I have found that certain laboratories provide more reliable results than others. Appendix One lists laboratories that I recommend.

BASIC TEST 1:
COMPLETE BLOOD CELL COUNT

This very common blood test measures various aspects of red and white blood cells, such as the number of red and white blood cells per cubic microliter of blood. A high number of a certain type of white blood cells (called eosinophils) can indicate allergy caused by environmental and food sensitivities, or parasites. These reactions can deplete your energy and nutrient reserves, and even affect your hormonal function. The size of your red blood cells can help determine whether there is a deficiency of either B_{12} or folic acid, which can cause all types of psychiatric symptoms, including mood swings. A reduced red blood cell size can indicate anemia (low iron), a common cause of fatigue. Treatment will vary depending on the results, but usually supplementation with vitamins or minerals is indicated.

Sometimes a B_{12} deficiency can even be the underlying cause of depression. For a year Francine, a fifty-five-year-old insurance executive, had been suffering from depression and frequent panic attacks, which began about the same time her only child left home for college. When Francine first came to see me, I attributed her symptoms to "empty nest syndrome" and an unsatisfying relationship with her husband. Over the course of several months, I prescribed one antidepressant, then another, as I combined her medications with weekly therapy sessions. Although her depression and panic attacks became somewhat less frequent, they did not disappear entirely.

After about one year of treatment, Francine paged me late at night while she was in the throes of a panic attack. She told me she was terrified and was having difficulty breathing. She said she felt dizzy and her heart was pounding so hard that it felt like it was going to explode. I talked with Francine and was unable to detect any reason for the attack. I told her to take a small increase in one of her medications and to call me if she didn't feel better in an hour. After I hung up the phone, though, a light went off in my head! I realized that the antidepressants should have completely eliminated the panic and prevented this attack. I knew there must be some hidden problem that I had missed.

I reviewed her chart, did some research, then brought Francine into the office for some blood tests. The tests revealed a deficiency in vitamin B_{12}. Further evaluation indicated that Francine's body was unable to absorb the vitamin. She had developed a condition called pernicious anemia. I gave her B_{12} injections with folic acid on a regular basis and monitored her closely for several weeks. She told me she no longer felt depressed and hadn't had a single panic attack since beginning the B_{12} therapy. Francine and I came to a joint decision that she should stop taking antidepressants.

Two years later Francine came back to my office with panic and depression. She had thought she didn't need to continue the B_{12} injections and had stopped them several months earlier. I restarted her on the B_{12} treatments, and her symptoms cleared immediately. Now, fourteen years later, she continues her B_{12} therapy and remains free from depression and panic attacks. (Francine referred her daughter to me for evaluation two years ago. She was seeing violent scenes in the bathroom mirror of her new home and was quite frightened. She also turned out to have a B_{12} deficiency, the treatment of which cleared her symptoms completely.)

Francine's case may sound like a testimonial you'd hear at a church revival meeting. But there is no magic or mysticism involved. Francine had an extreme deficiency in a nutrient needed by her brain cells to function normally. This deficiency was caused by a malfunction in her gastrointestinal tract that was preventing the absorption of vitamin B_{12} from the foods she ate. Francine's case is unusual in that her depression was caused solely by this nutritional deficiency. She does not illustrate the norm for most of my patients, the vast majority of whom still need to continue their use of antidepressants because their depression stems from a mixture of causes.

B₁₂ and Folic Acid Deficiencies

An entire volume could easily be written on vitamin B_{12}, folate, and psychiatric disorders. Both folate deficiency and B_{12} deficiency can present as a megaloblastic anemia, although multiple cases have been reported of deficiencies in the absence of macrocytosis—about 30 percent of cases in one report (S. D. Shovon et al., "The neuropsychiatry of megaloblastic anemia," *British Medical Journal* 281, 1980: 1036–42). In a more recent report (J. Lindenbaum et al., "Neuropsychiatric disorders caused by cobalamin deficiency in the absence of anemia or macrocytosis," *New England Journal of Medicine* 318, 1988: 1720–28), 28 percent of patients (40 out of 141) with neuropsychiatric symptoms showed no anemia or macrocytosis. According to *Cecil's Textbook of Medicine* (20th edition, edited by C. J. Bennett and F. Plum, Philadelphia, W. B. Saunders, 1996, p. 849), "Many patients with clinically confirmed cobalamin or folate deficiency have serum vitamin levels within the normal range."

Numerous studies have determined that patients with affective disorders have significantly lower levels of red blood cell folate, and a Baylor University Medical Center Proceeding (5, no. 4, 1992: 13–25) indicates that folate deficiency is more likely than B_{12} deficiency to appear as an affective disorder.

Thus, beyond the complete blood cell count, I strongly recommend testing the red blood cell folate as well as total fasting plasma homocysteine and urinary methylmalonic acid (MMA) in all patients. These tests add significantly to the frequency of diagnosis and treatment. The plasma homocysteine and urinary MMA are both functional tests of the methylation pathways. These two tests can be used to help separate out these deficiency states, since the MMA level is elevated in more than 95 percent of patients with clinically confirmed cobalamin deficiency but not folate deficiency. By contrast, homocysteine is elevated in both cobalamin and folate deficiency.

In the case of B_{12} deficiency, pernicious anemia with intrinsic factor deficiency must be ruled out. Treatment with both folate (1 milligram per day) and B_{12} (1 milligram by intramuscular injection three times weekly, in gradually decreasing frequency after one month, to once or twice monthly thereafter) must be undertaken immediately. In the case of folate deficiency alone, treatment with folic acid (2 to 4 milligrams per day) along with a B complex and following the homocysteine monthly until normal usually suffice. Treatment of both conditions usually results in improved outcome and reduction in psychiatric symptomatology.

I consider mild to moderate eosinophilia a good marker of immune activation, and there is a reasonable possibility that this immune activation is contributing to my patients' symptoms of fatigue, sluggishness, or cognitive dysfunction. Eosinophilia is well known to occur in several important diseases, including allergic disorders (most common cause), parasitic infections, inflammatory bowel disease, gastroenteritis, eczema, drug reactions, lymphomas, and, interestingly, cytokine infusions (M. E. Rothenberg, "Eosinophilia," *New England Journal of Medicine* 338, no. 22, 1998: 1592–1600). Cytokines are known to have effects on brain function (cytokine release from monocytes is suppressed by antidepressants), and immune activation can present as fatigue and decreased initiative. Ask your patient for a history of wheezing, eczema (also associated with zinc and essential fatty acid deficiencies), rhinitis, and food and chemical sensitivities. Inquire about travel to foreign countries (where helminthic infections are endemic) or the presence of a dog *(Toxocara canis),* as well as any drug ingestion.

In cases of mild eosinophilia (351 to 1500 cells per cubic millimeter of blood), the comprehensive digestive stool analysis (CDSA; see Note to Your Doctor, page 211), will help rule out parasitic infection. Elimination of allergens (food, chemical, environmental) will help improve patients' overall sense of energy, well-being, and probably cognitive and emotional function. Morphologic examination of a blood smear is a useful test if other causes of eosinophilia cannot be ruled out by the history and CDSA or in cases of moderate to severe eosinophilia (greater than 1500 cells per cubic millimeter). This must be interpreted by a hematologist.

BASIC TEST 2:
ESSENTIAL FATTY ACID ANALYSIS

My grandfather always called fish brain food. We thought he was nuts! Now scientists are confirming that my grandfather was smarter than we gave him credit for. In September of 1998 researchers at the National Institutes of Health held a conference entitled Workshop on Omega-3 Essential Fatty Acids. It is becoming apparent that insufficient intake of essential fatty acids—which are in high concentrations in fish—contributes to the development of some brain and nerve cell abnormalities, including ones that contribute to depression.

The essential fatty acid analysis test (EFA) measures the amounts and ratios of essential fatty acids in the red blood cell membrane. The test will determine if your levels of the two classes of essential fatty acids (omega-3 and omega-6) are in balance. Most of us have too little omega-3 (found in salmon, albacore tuna, mackerel, anchovies, sardines, lake trout, and Atlantic sturgeon) and too much omega-6 (found in nuts, meats, dairy products, and shellfish) and omega-9. Symptoms of low omega-3 levels include memory problems, mood swings, depression, frequent infections, numbness, and tingling of the extremities. (In fact, abnormalities of essential fatty acids are associated with at least sixty disorders!) High omega-6 levels can cause tissue inflammation, which can, through a variety of mechanisms, lower energy levels, reduce mental clarity, and cause depressed moods.

Treatment for low omega-3 levels is straightforward: Eat two to three fish meals a day (the varieties listed in the previous paragraph are best). If you can't eat that much fish, you can take a fish oil supplement. (I recommend a supplement called Zone Perfect fish oil, which includes other essential vitamins and contains no herbicides, pesticides, fungicides, or heavy metals—all substances that tend to accumulate in fat. It can be ordered by calling 800-233-3426.) Increase gradually to three 1000-milligram pills, three times a day, taken at the start of meals.

Note: Do not take more than the recommended dose of fish oil, since it can be toxic in high amounts and can interfere with blood clotting. Also, if you have problems digesting fats (indicated by belching or abdominal pain after a high-fat meal and yellow, foul-smelling stools that float), you may not be able to absorb the fish oil; you need to check with your doctor before taking a fish oil supplement.

NOTE TO YOUR DOCTOR

Essential Fatty Acid Analysis

According to Jerry Cott, Ph.D., of the National Institute of Mental Health, "Epidemiological studies in various countries and in the United States in the last century suggest that decreased omega-3 fatty acid consumption correlates with increasing rates of depression. There is evidence that deficiency of long-chain, omega-3 polyunsaturate may contribute to symptoms of schizophrenia, alcoholism, multiple sclerosis, and postpartum depression." Other researchers add bipolar disorder to the list. Whether the mechanism of action is mediated via oxidative injury, immune function and production of cytokines, or membrane-associated G-protein signal transduction is not known. Several double-blind placebo controlled studies support the use of essential fatty acid supplementation in treatment-resistant bipolar and schizophrenic disorders, and there is preliminary evidence of improvement in some tests of cognition.

Analysis of red blood cell membrane essential fatty acid concentration is the method used in most research and is available from Great Smokies Diagnostic Laboratory (800-522-4762). The test should be run with the patient in a fasting state. Results will indicate the levels of arachidonic acid, eicosapentaenoic acid (EPA), and docosahexaenoic acid (DHA), as well as a variety of ratios, including unsaturated to polyunsaturated fatty acids. A four-month trial of high-dose supplementation (9 grams per day) with a purified or organic form of fish oil is useful in those whose essential fatty acid analysis reveals low levels. Another source of essential fatty acids (EPA, DHA, and GLA), which has a very high absorption rate, is a water-soluble, microencapsulated powder called Omega Plex G, made and distributed by Interplexus, Inc. (800-875-0511). This can be taken once or twice daily in liquid. I recommend that the red blood cell essential fatty acid analysis be done before prescribing any fatty acids (and repeated in three-month intervals until a good balance is achieved), since different deficiencies and excesses exist in different individuals and require the use of different (organic) fatty acid supplements. Another excellent source of oils can be ordered by calling Udo Erasmus (604-731-4255).

BASIC TEST 3: MINERAL ANALYSIS

A mineral analysis, when performed by a reliable laboratory, will measure the levels of various minerals in your blood. *Nine out of ten of my patients have a deficiency in at least one of these trace minerals.*

Low levels of zinc are associated with treatment-resistant depression and can cause sexual dysfunction in men and low testosterone levels in both sexes. Low levels of magnesium can cause weakness and fatigue and may make it difficult to exercise. A deficiency in chromium, selenium, manganese, or vanadium can result in hypoglycemia, which can cause mood swings, irritability, and low energy. A deficiency in selenium can contribute to an underactive thyroid. All these deficiencies can mimic depression or the side effects of antidepressants.

High levels of aluminum have been associated with psychosis; cadmium with fatigue and anorexia; lead with adrenal dysfunction, anxiety, impaired concentration, depression, fatigue, memory impairment, and restlessness; and mercury with depression, emotional instability, fatigue, irritability, memory impairment, and psychosis.

Treatment may require a change in your diet and supplements specific to your imbalance. For instance, if you have low iron, take an iron supplement instead of a multimineral supplement. I don't favor these all-purpose supplements because the combination of minerals in one tablet can actually inhibit the absorption of the mineral you're lacking. For example, most multivitamins contain both zinc and chromium. However, absorption of chromium is decreased in the presence of zinc.

There are numerous interactions of this nature, so deficiencies are best corrected by targeted mineral supplementation.

NOTE TO YOUR DOCTOR

Mineral Analysis

Mineral and trace element deficiencies (quite common) or heavy metal toxicities (significantly less common) can play a major role in both treatment-resistant depression and what may appear to be side effects of antidepressants. Zinc deficiency impairs testosterone synthesis, which can mimic all the symptoms of depression as well as sexual dysfunction. Chromium and zinc are known to be cofactors for insulin, and chromium is known to be essential for the maintenance of normal glucose tolerance. Other suspected trace elements involved in glucose regulation include manganese, vanadium, and selenium (K. Kimura, "Role of essential trace elements in the disturbance of carbohydrate metabolism," *Nippon Rinsho*, 1996, 54(supplement 1): 79–84). Carbohydrate cravings are a common side effect of antidepressants and are common symptoms of certain types of depression as well.

It seems prudent when trying to manage side effects to rule out deficiencies of trace elements and excesses of heavy metals (particularly in treatment-resistant cases) that may contribute to or cause such symptoms. It is not prudent to supplement indiscriminately on the basis of the clinical picture alone, because there are multiple causes of such symptoms and excess levels of these minerals can be toxic.

In my experience patients from different areas of the country tend to have different deficiencies, and I suspect that variations in soil and food preferences may be the cause. As usual a good history can help confirm a suspicion of heavy metal toxicity (such was the case in an assembly-line worker in a poultry-processing plant, who had markedly high levels of lead and cadmium, along with the classic symptoms of these metal toxicities).

Mineral analysis can be performed via blood and urine or hair samples. Hair has the potential of being a very useful tool to complement blood and urine analyses (T. H. Maugh, "Hair: a diagnostic tool to complement blood serum and urine," *Science,* 1978, 202: 1271–73; D. W. Jenkins and J. A. Santolucito, *Biological Monitoring of Toxic Trace Metals,* vol. 1: *Biological Monitoring and Surveillance,* Las Vegas, Environmental Monitoring Systems Laboratory, Office of Research and Development, U.S. Environmental Protection Agency, 1980; and S. C. Foo et al., "Metals in hair as biological indices for exposure," *International Archives of Occupational and Environmental Health*, 1993, 65: S83–S86). However, one of the main advantages of hair sampling is also its main disadvantage; that is, its easy accessibility, which also contributes to contamination problems. Great Smokies Diagnostic Laboratory has now established a laboratory that they claim is free from contaminants. A patient submitting a hair sample must prepare for three weeks by using only Johnson's baby shampoo to limit the contamination from shampoos. This may turn out to be a useful, relatively inexpensive screening tool, particularly for heavy metal exposure, since hair (unlike blood and urine) is a tissue in which heavy metals are sequestered and therefore reflects long-term exposure to these metals, which also tend to be sequestered in internal tissues and organs (for instance, bone, brain, and kidneys).

In most cases of carbohydrate cravings and intolerance, sexual dysfunction, fatigue, weight gain, and mood disturbances (when I do not suspect a heavy metal toxicity), I prefer to screen for trace elements using red blood cells, plasma, and urine. The Bay Area Laboratory Co-operative (BALCO, 800-777-7122) is a reliable lab, with the best quality control I can find. I have used local laboratories; however, results in the same patient have been quite erratic (in two samples from one patient, a plasma manganese was reported with a difference of ten times the value!). Reports from BALCO come back with recommendations; however, I suggest an element-by-element review with your own determination of appropriate supplementation. Given the standard error allowed on their testing (plus or minus 10 percent), I supplement the patient's diet with any element that is in the lowest tenth to fifteenth percentile of the normal range.

Digestion Self-Evaluation

1. Do you have frequent heartburn?

2. Do you feel bloated or have prolonged fullness or heaviness in your stomach after eating?

3. Do you belch frequently, or have a lot of gas?

4. Do you have chronic constipation or diarrhea?

5. Do you have tan-colored, foul-smelling stools that float?

These are all signs that you may have some malfunctioning in your body's digestion or absorption of food.

DIGESTIVE ABNORMALITIES

Keep this important fact in mind: *You can be eating all the right foods in all the right ratios, but you may still have nutritional deficiencies if your food is not being properly processed and absorbed by your digestive system.* A host of maladies can cause this kind of problem. You may not have enough acid or digestive enzymes in your stomach, or you may have too few "friendly" bacteria that break down food in your intestines. If the ecosystem in your gut is out of balance, certain nutrients will never make it to your brain, and other molecules that shouldn't make it into your system might slip through.

Let's say your gut cannot break down the protein you eat into essential amino acids, which are the building blocks of neurotransmitters. Your brain's serotonin-releasing cells will "sit idle" as they wait for the delivery of amino acids that never come. This sets off a chain reaction: Your body can't get the raw materials to your brain cells, so your brain cannot keep the rest of your body (including your digestive system) in good balance. Without a proper supply of brain chemicals, you may feel depressed, anxious, or tired, and have trouble concentrating. You also may feel out of sorts and moody because your antidepressants can't work without the necessary neurotransmitters. In fact, several recent studies have documented that people who lack the amino acids tryptophan and tyrosine are at greater risk of suffering a depressive relapse while taking antidepressants.

A clear example of how poor digestion can interfere with the use of antidepressants is Ned, a very bright fifteen-year-old boy whom I recently treated for depression. Ned's primary-care doctor had prescribed Zoloft, but Ned had not responded to this treatment and was sluggish and tired all the time. Ned's mother complained that he spent hours zoning out in front of the TV and would barely respond when she asked him questions.

During my evaluation, I learned that Ned had been experiencing frequent gas and diarrhea, especially when he ate meat or dairy foods. A blood test of his essential fatty acid levels revealed that Ned's omega-3 fatty acids were very low. Further testing showed that Ned had both not been eating enough omega-3-rich fish and had a problem absorbing these fats from his diet.

Ned told me he was willing to try my program. I first put him on the Five-Day Jump Start, and he immediately felt more energy. We worked together to improve his diet, and he slowly gave up all caffeine, sugar, and refined starches, such as bagels and white bread. We found ways to work more protein and fat into his diet and normalized his digestion through supplements. I recommended that he eat two fish meals a day. And I prescribed fish oil supplements, as well as zinc and chromium (since he was found to be significantly deficient in both minerals). Ned also made an effort to increase his exercise. Over the next few months the antidepressants began to have beneficial effects, and Ned told me that he no longer felt depressed and was actually feeling happier. He decided to join a computer club at school, the first time he had ever taken part in an after-school activity.

GETTING TESTED FOR DIGESTIVE ABNORMALITIES

I recommend a test called a comprehensive digestive stool analysis (CDSA). Stool tests are pretty routine (although not for psychiatrists) and require you to take a kit home and collect samples of your stool.

The CDSA, a particularly thorough version of the standard stool test, looks for evidence of maldigestion of fat and protein; pancreatic function; abnormal bacteria, yeast, and parasites; metabolic markers; and blood. This test is extremely helpful to ascertain if the food you eat is being properly digested and absorbed into your body, and what might be causing any difficulties. Your doctor should use the CDSA performed by Great Smokies Diagnostic Laboratory (see Appendix One) because their results on this test are reliable and thorough.

TREATMENT FOR DIGESTIVE ABNORMALITIES

Treatment varies depending on what the lab report shows. Your stool may contain evidence of a maldigestion of protein, an inability to absorb fats, a low level of good bacteria that aid in digestion, the presence of parasites, or high levels of yeast or abnormal bacteria. I've outlined some of the more common problems found, but I encourage you to work with your doctor and the lab itself to develop a specific plan for you.

Maldigestion: If your results show excessive amounts of undigested foods like meat or vegetables, you may not be chewing your food well or may have too little stomach acid or inadequate pancreatic enzymes. If you tend to be a fast eater, give yourself smaller portions at a time and chew more slowly. Also, drink at least one eight-ounce glass of water with every meal. If you feel bloated after you eat, belch frequently, and are constipated, you may be producing inadequate stomach acid, which can be associated with vitamin B_{12} deficiency and may result from taking antacids on a regular basis. An immediately effective remedy is an over-the-counter stomach acid pill called betaine hydrochloride, which is found in most nutrition or health-food stores. Take one capsule (approximately 600 milligrams) in the middle of the meal with a full glass of water. You must take the capsule *in the middle of the meal* with a full glass of water because it can burn the lining of your stomach if you take it before or after eating. Take one pill with every meal (though not with light snacks). If you're having a particularly heavy meal, you might need to take two capsules or more to bring full relief from your gas symptoms and ensure full digestion. Check with your doctor before taking a stomach acid pill, because the pill could be dangerous if you have an ulcer or esophogeal reflux.

If your lab results also show insufficient levels of pancreatic enzymes, you may need to take a pancreatic enzyme supplement, available in most health-food stores. Check with your doctor to make sure this treatment will be safe and effective for you.

Inability to absorb fats: If your gastrointestinal tract is unable to digest fats properly, nerve cells in your brain are likely to be lacking adequate amounts of the fat-soluble vitamins A, D, E, and K, as well as the omega-3 fatty acids, which are necessary for normal brain function. Treatment can be complicated, and the cause of the problem needs to be determined. I usually refer my patients to a gastroenterologist to have their gallbladder function evaluated. Discuss with your doctor whether you need to have further testing.

Low levels of "good" bacteria: A proper amount of "good" bacteria (lactobacillus and bifidobacillus) in your intestines is vital for your body to manufacture certain vitamins, like folic acid, biotin, pantothenic acid, riboflavin, pyridoxine, vitamin B_{12}, and vitamin K from the nutrients you eat and absorb. A deficiency in any of these vitamins could cause an imbalance in your body, resulting in an array of symptoms that mimic depression, fatigue, anxiety, and even, in advanced cases, sexual dysfunction. You can get your levels of good bacteria back to where they should be by taking regular doses of UltraFlora Plus, DF (Dairy Free), which is found in health-food stores or can be ordered from Metagenics (800-647-6100). Take one-half teaspoon in a glass of water two to three times a day on an empty stomach. Continue treatment until you have finished two bottles. After that, eating a high-quality yogurt with active mixed cultures is a good way to maintain the population of these beneficial bacteria.

NOTE TO YOUR DOCTOR

Treatment for Digestive Abnormalities

The Comprehensive Digestive Stool Analysis (CDSA) must be interpreted individually and appropriate interventions chosen on a case-by-case basis. An acceptable approach to treating digestive abnormalities (not caused by other medical conditions, such as gallbladder disease, liver disease, ulcers, and so on) is to follow a medically proven program created by Dr. Jeffrey Bland (founder of HealthComm International, Inc., a functional medicine research company in Gig Harbor, Washington) called the Four R Program. The Four R's are

1. *Remove:* Eliminate any abnormal bacteria, yeast, or parasites from the intestinal tract, as well as offending foods (using history and the food elimination diet). The CDSA comes with sensitivity testing for any pathological agents found.

2. *Replace:* Supplement with digestive factors or enzymes that may be secreted in insufficient amounts, such as hydrochloric acid, gastric pepsin, pancreatic enzymes (e.g., trypsin, chymotrypsin, lipase, amylase), bile, intestinal enzymes (e.g., lactase), and fiber.

3. *Reinoculate:* Reintroduce the "friendly bacteria" *Lactobacillus* species *(acidophilus, bulgaricus,* and *thermophilus),* as well as bifidobacteria species *(bifidus, infantis,* and so on). Normal gut flora produce at least six essential nutrients necessary for normal nervous system function (folic acid, biotin, pantothenic acid, riboflavin, pyridoxine, and cobalamin). (P. A. Mackowiak, "The normal bacterial flora," *New England Journal of Medicine* 307, 1982: 83–93.) The use of fructooligosaccharides has been shown to promote the growth of these beneficial bacteria. I frequently use a product called UltraFlora Plus, DF (dairy free) produced by Metagenics: one-half teaspoon in warm water, twice daily until the patient has used two bottles.

4. *Repair:* Provide appropriate nutritional support for restoration and maintenance of the gastrointestinal mucosa. In this last step of the program, I frequently use UltraClear Sustain (made by Metagenics), a hypoallergenic rice-based product that contains a number of factors necessary for the repair process.

Liver Self-Evaluation

1. Do you require unusually small amounts of medications?

2. Are you very sensitive to the effects of caffeine?

3. Are you sensitive to perfumes, exhaust fumes, or strong odors?

4. Are you sensitive to foods containing sulfites (wine, dried fruits, salad bar vegetables)?

5. Do you feel uncomfortable after eating foods with garlic or onions?

6. Do you drink alcohol on a daily basis?

If you answer yes to any one of these questions, you may be having difficulty metabolizing and eliminating your medications, as well as other chemicals to which you are exposed. If this is the case, I suggest you have a liver detoxification profile done. This test, performed by Great Smokies Diagnostic Laboratory (see Appendix One), can define to a reasonable degree the pathways that are not functioning properly. Often the activity level in the various pathways can be corrected, resulting in improved ability to tolerate antidepressants, decreased fatigue, and reduction of "brain fog" and cognitive dysfunction.

MEDICATION INTOLERANCE

About 10 to 15 percent of people have difficulty tolerating normal antidepressant doses because of severe side effects such as excessive sedation, lethargy, difficulty in thinking clearly, headache, and nausea, among others. While it's true that some people are genetically wired to metabolize drugs slowly, some people with an intolerance to antidepressants have nutritional deficits that prevent their livers from efficiently metabolizing the drugs.

If you have difficulty tolerating antidepressants, try a food-based product called UltraClear Plus, available in health-food stores or by calling Metagenics (800-647-6100). This very healthy, low-allergen product is made from a rice-based protein supplemented with various vitamins, minerals, and amino acids and is designed specifically to help your liver function at optimal capacity. Some of my patients who have difficulty tolerating antidepressants—even at low doses—have been helped by using this product. Start by mixing one-quarter scoop of powder in eight ounces of water twice a day. Gradually increase over a period of two weeks to two scoops of powder in eight ounces of water twice daily.

There are a number of simple measures you can take to improve your liver's ability to detoxify efficiently.

1. Avoid foods that are likely to contain chemicals or to which you might be sensitive. Food sensitivities can be determined by following the food elimination diet on page 224.
2. Drink plenty of clean water.
3. Take in good amounts of high-quality protein, and avoid caffeine and alcohol (as you will by following the Fundamentals).
4. Take the liver detoxification profile test and supplement with the nutrients necessary to improve the function of the imbalanced pathways.

NOTE TO YOUR DOCTOR

Treating Liver Intolerance to Medication

The liver detoxifies xenobiotics (substances that are foreign to the body, whether of external origin or metabolic intermediates, and by-products of foods or drugs that are inadequately detoxified or eliminated) by a two-phase process. In the first phase, a large group of isoenzymes such as the Cytochrome P450 family act on antidepressants via oxidation, reduction, hydrolysis, and dehalogenation to create intermediate compounds with different biological activities than the parent compound. These intermediate compounds are then rendered metabolically inert and ready for elimination by conjugation reactions such as sulfation, glutathione conjugation, methylation, glucoronidation, acetylation, or amino acid conjugation.

Imbalances in these liver detoxification systems can lead to increased side effects via a number of mechanisms, as well as to cognitive dysfunction and fatigue. As an example, caffeine is metabolized by the Cytochrome P450 1A2 isoenzyme. If this system is overactive, levels of the antidepressant metabolite norfluoxetine could be reduced. If, on the other hand, a patient is placed on fluoxetine and then decides to drink caffeine (which is cleared by the 1A2 isoenzyme), the norfluoxetine metabolite would have inhibited the activity of this enzyme to the point that there would be increased sensitivity to caffeine, with "side effects" of insomnia, agitation, and so on.

In other cases, the patient's P450 system could be induced by xenobiotics, and the second phase of detoxification could be slow due to metabolic deficiencies. The result would be a bottleneck effect, with a buildup of toxic intermediate substances producing side effects.

In practical terms, there is much we do not know about these detoxification systems, but research is advancing quickly. We do know that phase one reactions require cofactors such as a number of the B vitamins (B_2, B_3, folate, B_{12}), branched chain amino acids, glutathione, minerals, flavonoids, and phospholipids, and that these phase one reactions produce reactive intermediates that can cause side effects, as well as free radicals and tissue damage. Protective strategies include the use of nutrients (such as vitamins A, C, and E, selenium, garlic, onions, cruciferous vegetables, manganese, zinc, and copper) and provision of phase two "raw materials," such as amino acids (e.g., glycine, taurine, methionine), N-acetylcysteine, and so on.

I recommend a detoxification profile be performed on patients who have answered in the affirmative to any of the self-evaluation questions on page 213. The test report will be accompanied by an interpretation guide, and further guidelines are available from the laboratory.

If this is not feasible, I suggest that the patient begin using a product made by Metagenics (800-647-6100) called UltraClear

Plus. Have the patient start with a small dose (one-quarter scoop twice daily in water) and work up as tolerated to the full dose (two scoops twice daily). This product provides a very reasonable level of the above-mentioned nutrients and has been useful to a significant number of my patients who answered the self-evaluation questions in the affirmative and who were suffering from fatigue, "brain fog," and intolerance of antidepressants.

A good monograph on this subject for clinicians, "Detoxification: A Clinical Monograph," can be ordered from the Institute for Functional Medicine in Gig Harbor, Washington (800-228-0622).

HYPOGLYCEMIA

The control of blood sugar within a normal range is a very complex process, which involves multiple chemicals (epinephrine, insulin, glucagon, cortisol) and minerals (chromium, selenium, manganese, and vanadium). With careful questioning I have found that about 50 percent of my patients experience symptoms of hypoglycemia. Hypoglycemia contributes to the weight gain caused by antidepressants.

What exactly is hypoglycemia? It is an intermittent but usually long-term condition that causes blood-sugar levels to fall below the normal range necessary for optimal functioning of the brain and body. Your body can respond to the early stages of hypoglycemia by causing intense cravings for sweets and starches. This is your body signaling your brain that you need more glucose in your bloodstream—*now!* Once your body is in this state, you may either feed these cravings with carbohydrates or drink something with caffeine—which temporarily causes a release of adrenaline, which raises your blood sugar. If you don't respond, you will feel woozy, irritable, or nervous. Most people take a quick sugar fix. This causes temporary relief by increasing blood sugar, but it also increases the output of insulin and cortisol, both of which lead to weight gain and further blood-sugar problems. It's a vicious cycle that quickly spins out of control.

If you're hypoglycemic, your pancreas gradually becomes ill-equipped to handle foods high in sugar or other simple carbohydrates. These are foods that have a high glycemic index, which means your

Hypoglycemia Self-Evaluation

1. If you miss a meal or go more than three or four hours without eating, do you experience any of the following symptoms: irritable, restless, jittery, dizzy, nauseous, light-headed, sweaty, trouble concentrating, headache?

2. If so, are these symptoms alleviated by food?

3. Do you frequently crave sugar, cakes, cookies, sweets, or alcohol?

4. Have you gained ten pounds or more since beginning antidepressants?

These are all signs that you may have a condition known as hypoglycemia, or low blood sugar.

---

body rapidly breaks them down into glucose and shuttles this glucose into your bloodstream to give you instant energy. Eventually, your pancreas responds too forcefully, by releasing too much insulin to help your cells use the glucose in your blood. So instead of giving you a sustained amount of energy, your blood-sugar levels spike temporarily before plunging again. Any excess sugar not used by your cells gets carted away to be stored as fat—which is why you gain weight. The more you feed your sugar cravings, the less efficient your body becomes at using the sugar. As a result, you feel more intense hunger, which makes you eat more sugar, which causes you to gain weight. Starting to get the picture?

When you bring antidepressants to the mix (with the exception of Serzone and Wellbutrin), you frequently add at least one or two other mechanisms to the weight gain dilemma. All antidepressants that affect serotonin initially cause an increase in serotonin availability. This reduces appetite and contributes to weight loss (which is why the makers of Prozac, Eli Lilly, initially considered marketing it to help with weight reduction). Eventually, however, for most people, the nerve cells adjust to this state, and the net effect can be less (but more efficient) serotonin activity, resulting in increased appetite. In addition to this mechanism, many antidepressants can have an antihistamine effect, which in and of itself may cause weight gain.

The bottom line is that when you add the hypoglycemic drive to eat simple carbohydrates to the serotonin and antihistamine mechanisms, you have a prescription for serious weight gain—and serious loss of self-esteem. Not only have you gained twenty pounds but you can't seem to get a handle on your sugar cravings!

DIAGNOSIS OF AND TREATMENT FOR HYPOGLYCEMIA

If you have any of the signs of hypoglycemia, you need to discuss your symptoms with your doctor. Before your appointment, keep a food diary for a week. Write down everything you ate, how you felt right after eating, and whether you experienced any symptoms (fatigue, wooziness, irritability, and so on) one to three hours later. Keep a record of your food cravings and how you dealt with them.

Take this food diary to your doctor. It will be a basis of your diagnosis. Unfortunately, there is no reliable test to confirm whether you have hypoglycemia. (Many doctors perform a glucose tolerance test, in which the peaks and valleys of your blood-sugar levels are measured for several hours after drinking a high sugar beverage. I've found that this test frequently enough misses clinically confirmed cases of hypoglycemia. For this reason, I don't perform it on my patients.)

If you do have signs of hypoglycemia, following the nutrition plan will help get the condition under control. Forgoing sugar, alcohol, caffeine, and refined carbohydrates will help stabilize your blood-sugar levels very rapidly. Eating an increased amount of protein will give you sustained energy. Replenishing your minerals will be critical.

Realize, though, that when you begin the nutrition plan you may not feel well as your body adjusts to less sugar. The first three or four days are the hardest: Many of my patients report feeling weak, dizzy, tired, and moody. After this initial stage, though, your energy will rebound, your depression will lift, and you'll be free from your cravings. By six weeks your taste buds and preferences will have changed so much that you will be surprised you once thought those sweet foods tasted so good. You'll probably also notice that your clothes are looser as you begin to lose weight and retain less fluid. On the flip side, if you cheat a little and sneak some cookies or ice cream, you'll see that your hypoglycemic symptoms will quickly return, and your taste buds and preferences will not change.

You also need to make four additional modifications to your eating habits to keep hypoglycemia at bay:

1. *Eat five or six small balanced meals a day.* More frequent meals will keep your blood-sugar levels stable and should prevent hypoglycemic symptoms.

2. *Be sure these meals or snacks contain the right carbohydrate-to-protein ratio.* Snacks should have at least 7 grams of protein for every 10 grams of carbohydrates. Read the food labels. Or, if there is no label to read, eyeball the food. The protein (meat, fish, turkey, and so on) portion should be slightly more than one-third the volume of the meal, with the other two-thirds being carbohydrate. Snacks that are balanced will help reduce sugar cravings and keep your appetite under control. Some great balanced snacks include a handful of nuts with some fresh fruit, a cup of vanilla yogurt sprinkled with wheat germ, cottage cheese on a rye cracker.

3. *Avoid artificial sweeteners.* No, they aren't sugar, but they can contribute to sugar cravings. If your body is used to getting something sweet, it will continue to crave sugar.

4. *Learn to recognize the difference between fatigue and hunger.* We often gravitate toward sweet foods thinking they will give us an energy boost when the real problem is fatigue and stress. This depletion usually is associated with cravings toward the end of the day (when you are most tired) or after a night or more of inadequate sleep. Five minutes of meditation or simple relaxation will usually alleviate the problem for a while. Catching up on your nighttime sleep will also help a lot.

NOTE TO YOUR DOCTOR

Diagnosis and Treatment of Hypoglycemia

In my experience, antidepressants can cause or worsen hypoglycemia in many patients. Antidepressants may increase appetite via histamine or serotonergic mechanisms (possibly via the 5-HT$_2$c receptor). Initially, with the serotonergic reuptake inhibition caused by the antidepressant, you will note decreased appetite in your patients. As the postsynaptic serotonergic receptors downregulate in response to the increased serotonin output, the net effect is often a decrease in serotonergic activity, probably in the serotonergic neurons that run from the raphe (midbrain) to the hypothalamus. Decreased serotonergic activity in this pathway is associated with increased eating. Serzone is unique in that it increases serotonergic output from the presynaptic neuron but blocks the 5-HT$_2$c receptors, so there is no increased serotonergic activity at these receptors and perhaps then no alteration in the raphe-hypothalamic serotonin pathway.

Patients who are clinically hypoglycemic already have a tendency to overeat (independent of the serotonergic and antihistamine drives), particularly carbohydrates. Intervening in this mechanism will help reduce this contribution to weight gain, which occurs at least in part via elevated glucose levels, with gradual insulin resistance, increased insulin output, consequent increased levels of cortisol, and sequestration of glucose in adipose tissue.

I don't put much stock in the glucose tolerance test because of its high rate of false negatives. A far more reliable method is to have your patients keep a written record of what they've eaten and when they experience the onset of symptoms (such as irritability, moodiness, fatigue). They should also note the effect of a high-carbohydrate snack on their symptoms. I keep a box of fruit cookies in my office and offer a few to fasting patients whom I suspect are experiencing low blood-sugar levels at the time of their appointments. I then see if they feel any better.

If you suspect hypoglycemia based on history, you can try

putting the patient on the Five-Day Jump Start to confirm whether dietary intervention will help improve symptoms. If the patient closely follows the plan and notes significant improvement, you should consider the diagnosis of hypoglycemia reasonably likely. Treating the hypoglycemia with frequent meals balanced with low glycemic index carbohydrates as well as high-quality protein generally has a very beneficial impact on the patient's energy, weight, and mood.

In addition, you should perform a mineral profile, since low chromium, vanadium, and possibly manganese and selenium levels are clearly associated with glucose intolerance. If the patient's mineral profile comes back with low or borderline low levels of these minerals, I recommend supplementing fairly aggressively, rechecking the levels in two to three months. Vanadium has been associated with mood-altering properties, but I have not had the occasion to intervene with this mineral in any of my patients. Chromium can be used in doses of 150 to 200 micrograms three times a day. Patients need to be monitored because toxicity can occur, manifested by dermatitis, gastrointestinal ulcers, and kidney and liver disease.

FOOD SENSITIVITIES OR ALLERGIES

I had been treating a forty-five-year-old woman named Tina for depression with the antidepressant Pamelor. Although Tina was responding reasonably well to the medication, she had become increasingly anxious about her arthritis. She told me her hands and fingers were stiff, sometimes even numb, and she felt pain and stiffness in her left shoulder and her ankles. At times she would spend most of her day fixating on her pain, and she had convinced herself that the arthritis would one day cripple her.

Rather than giving Tina a prescription for tranquilizers to ease her anxiety, I convinced her to go on a food elimination diet, since certain foods may cause inflammation that can aggravate arthritis. I also knew that food allergies or sensitivities could be associated with the anxiety and depression she was feeling.

Tina avoided certain foods for a few weeks, and she called me to

Food Sensitivity and Allergy Self-Evaluation

1. Are you sensitive to any foods?

2. Do you suffer from skin problems, hay fever, asthma, or frequent colds or sinus infections?

3. Do you have dark circles under your eyes?

4. Do you have frequent rashes, headaches, congestion, or other types of allergic reactions to strong chemicals like perfume, household cleaners, detergents?

5. Do you have joint stiffness, headaches, muscle aches, or arthritis?

6. Do you have trouble thinking clearly ("brain fog")?

7. Do you get bloated (puffiness in abdomen, hands, or feet) easily?

8. Do your moods swing rapidly—from minute to minute, or hour to hour—without any real reason?

These are all signs that your body may be sensitive to one or more foods in your diet.

---

report that her ankles felt "98 percent better" and that her shoulders and hands felt "80 percent better." More important, she told me that she was no longer afraid that her arthritis was going to get worse. As she later confided, a major source of her "background worry," which she had never really discussed openly, was that she would become debilitated and unable to work.

I knew that one of the foods Tina was avoiding must be the offending culprit. The question was, which one? To find out, I instructed her to reintroduce certain foods into her diet one at a time to determine if any would make her arthritis worse. Tina discovered that every time she ate shellfish, chocolate, and sugars, her joints would ache over the next few days. She has since limited her intake of these foods to no more than a serving or two a week, and she has noticed a dramatic improvement in how she feels.

"Now that I'm nearly free of pain," Tina wrote me, "I sleep very well, my energy level is high, and, in general, I feel relaxed and happy. My feet have been totally free from pain and numbness, except occasionally when I go off the diet on weekends."

Margie, a forty-one-year-old advertising executive, came to me with extremely high levels of anxiety and intermittent depression related to a separation from her abusive husband a year earlier. I prescribed Paxil, which worked reasonably well, relieving all but some intermittent symptoms that were bothersome but not dramatically detracting from her life. In discussing her general state of health with me one day, she mentioned that she was having numerous skin problems. That was when I suggested the food elimination diet.

The result was remarkable. Margie came back to see me three months later feeling better than she had in years. Her skin problems had cleared, but even more notable to me was the fact that her anxiety and depressive symptoms were totally absent—for the first time in as long as she could remember. In disbelief I asked Margie about other changes in her life that might have accounted for her dramatic recovery. Was there a new relationship? No. Nothing except her diet had changed. I have been surprised again and again by such dramatic improvements in my patients, since my training had not indicated any such connection could be possible.

How is your mood affected by food sensitivities? A great deal is still unknown about these mechanisms, and many clinicians (I was one of them) do not give the food-mood connection much credence. However, once I saw the clinical evidence that eliminating certain foods in the diet can affect psychiatric symptoms, I was forced to do some research. Again, as with my research on the salivary tests of adrenal gland function, I found that there are well-established and accepted scientific facts that had not trickled down to most clinicians.

Here's what I discovered:

As the food you eat is digested and then absorbed, your immune system monitors the incoming chemicals and nutrients. When the immune cells are activated by an offending agent, they release cytokines, which, among other functions, provide your brain with a "chemical status report" on whether there is immune activity against an offending food or chemical. Your brain responds by altering its production of a number of neurochemicals (serotonin, norepinephrine, acetylcholine) that affect neurotransmission as well as gastrointestinal, hormone, and immune system function. Together with the cytokines, these changes can cause headaches, fuzziness of thinking, lack of energy, anxiety, extremely rapid mood shifts, or irritability. You might also experience a wide variety of physical complaints, including but not limited to abdominal pains, diarrhea, constipation, bloating, or joint aches.

If you have an *allergy* to certain foods or chemicals, you may have an immediate reaction to the offending food—within seconds, or up to an hour later—sneezing, wheezing, trouble breathing, throat swelling, hives, severe stomach pain, irritability. Far more common, though, is a delayed reaction caused by a food *sensitivity*. This reaction can occur up to three days after you have eaten the food! For this reason, pinpointing the exact food that caused your reaction takes some detective work. Are you feeling drained because of the pizza you ate last night, or the pasta with clam sauce you ate three days ago?

Treatment for Food Sensitivities: The Food Elimination Diet

Uncovering the foods you're sensitive to can be a challenging task. Unfortunately, there's no perfectly reliable blood test available to determine which foods are the offenders. I prefer to use the food elimination approach first, since it is less costly and very healthy. If, afterward, there is still a suspicion of food sensitivity or chemical sensitivity, appropriate testing can be done, although detective work is still the mainstay of diagnosis and treatment.

In certain cases, when the food elimination diet is too overwhelming for people, I use Immunolab's IgG food sensitivity testing (see Appendix One). While not perfect, in that some nonoffending foods seem to be identified, this test does quite frequently pinpoint the offending foods.

Here's my suggested protocol for ferreting out food allergies.

1. First, follow the balanced nutrition plan for a month. You may be able to avoid foods that you're sensitive to just by eliminating caffeine, chocolate, wheat flour (and things made from wheat flour), and sugar—which are among the most common offenders.

2. If you are still experiencing symptoms of inflammation after a month on the nutrition plan (see the self-evaluation on page 222), go on the food elimination diet. This is a standard and very healthy (but extremely restrictive) eating plan that many allergists hand out to their patients to identify foods that may be causing symptoms. The food elimination diet requires you to avoid the foods most commonly associated with food sensitivities. It requires planning; you need to map out your meals and read food labels carefully to ensure that none of the foods you eat contains ingredients you're supposed to avoid. For instance, potato chips may contain soybean oil, and certain salad dressings may contain cheese.

3. Before you go on the food elimination diet, make a list of *all* your symptoms: physical (fatigue, weight gain, trouble with sexual arousal, joint aches, upset stomach, sinus problems, and so on), emotional (mood swings, irritability, anxiety, depression), and mental (trouble concentrating, difficulty with memory, brain fog).

4. Rate each symptom on a scale of 1 to 4 (1 = occasional and mild, 2 = occasional and bothersome, 3 = frequent and mild, and 4 = frequent and bothersome). Tape your symptom list to the inside of the back cover of this book so it doesn't get lost, or get a separate notebook for this part of the program.

5. Stay on the food elimination diet for at least four and preferably six weeks. (Body tissues generally take six weeks to heal completely from minor injuries.) At the end of that time, retake the quiz on page 222 and rate your physical, emotional, and mental symptoms again, checking the list you made in Step 4.

The Food Elimination Diet

Eliminate all foods from the following categories.

1. Milk and all dairy products (cheese, yogurt, sour cream, butter, whey)
2. Wheat products (bread, cakes, wheat bran, and anything made with flour)*
3. Sugars (refined sugar, glucose, fructose, maltodextrin, maple syrup, honey, corn syrup, molasses, modified cornstarch)*
4. Citrus fruits and all processed fruit juices (unless freshly squeezed) and foods sweetened with fruit juice*
5. Corn (corn syrup, modified cornstarch, corn chips, popcorn)
6. Nuts (particularly peanuts) and soybeans and soy products (any food containing soybean oil, tofu, or soy sauce)
7. Caffeinated foods and beverages (coffee, colas, chocolate)*
8. Tomatoes and tomato-based products (tomato sauce, ketchup, tomato paste), as well as potatoes and eggplant
9. Foods containing yeast (breads that rise, beer and wine)
10. Beef and pork
11. Shellfish
12. Eggs and products made with eggs (for instance, mayonnaise, Caesar salad dressing)

*Note: You should be avoiding these foods already if you're following the balanced nutrition plan.

Foods You Can Eat

Turkey, chicken, and duck
Fish (other than shellfish)
Lamb
Whole grains (except wheat and corn)—rice, barley, oats, rye
Lentils, beans, and other legumes
Fresh fruits (except citrus and strawberries) and vegetables
Seeds (for example, sunflower seeds)
Goat milk and goat milk products

Sample Menu

Note: Eat as much as you wish. Just keep the balance of protein and carbohydrates appropriate. See if you can eat to fullness, an often brief signal from your brain. Then, take a few deep breaths and wrap the remaining food up for your snack in a couple of hours.

Breakfast

Carbohydrate: Bowl of oatmeal (slow-cooked)
or
Mixed-grain muesli (for instance, barley and oats with diced apples and cinnamon) cooked with rice milk
or
1 large piece of fresh fruit
Protein: Several slices of smoked salmon, turkey, herring, or white-fish
Spring water

Lunch

Salade Niçoise (1 can of tuna—protein—mixed with olive or flaxseed oil and lemon juice, or an olive oil–vinaigrette dressing. Serve with mixed greens, capers, and green beans.)
Spring water
If you prefer a simpler meal, try several slices of turkey with mustard on a rice cake, a piece of fresh fruit, and a glass of cold spring water.

Dinner

Cup of chicken soup
Grilled chicken, turkey, or fish
Rice and lentils (cook in chicken or vegetable broth)
Slice of melon
Spring water

After four to six weeks on this diet, you're ready to reintroduce the foods you eliminated.

Introduce one food category per week, and eat this food in frequent "doses" of three servings a day, for two days. (Remember to maintain your balance of proteins and carbohydrates. If you fail to maintain the balance, you will feel sluggish and misinterpret the sluggishness as a food sensitivity.) Reassess your symptoms every day for five days following your reintroduction of the food group. Write down any physical, emotional, or mental changes that you've experienced or suspect you have experienced since reintroducing the food. If you suspect you have a sensitivity to a certain food, eliminate it again for a week, then reintroduce it as a test.

Once you have identified the foods that cause you problems, you may eliminate them completely, or you may have them occasionally in small amounts. Understand, though, that inflammation is one common denominator of many diseases (such as heart disease and Alzheimer's disease), and the inflammatory response to these foods can contribute, over the long term, to the development of the diseases you are genetically predisposed to. Unfortunately, the foods we tend to prefer are often the foods we tend to be most sensitive to. Work toward a sensible balance once you have identified your food sensitivities.

Helpful Hint: You'll find that some foods fall into two or more categories. For instance, bread falls into the yeast and flour categories. When introducing a new category into your diet, try to include only those foods that fall into one category or into a category that you've already introduced. For instance, if you start by reintroducing foods containing flour, eat two or three servings a day of pasta or matzoh, which contain no yeast, instead of bread.

CHAPTER TEN

Reclaiming a Healthy Sex Drive

* * *

SIGMUND FREUD ROCKED the Western world when he identified libido (Eros) as the "life force." He theorized that our sex drive is behind everything that motivates us: in disguised form it propels us out of bed in the morning and motivates us to work and succeed and connect with people. Freud introduced the concept of the pleasure principle as a constant drive that fuels a lifetime of craving and fulfillment.

In Freud's view (and while I don't subscribe to many of his theories, I believe he was right on the money in this regard), sex is the litmus test of our capacity to enjoy life *fully*—our work, our relationships, ourselves. *Just as depression is closely linked with the inability to experience pleasure, a healthy sex drive and a fulfilling, well-balanced sex life are critical barometers of overall mental and physical well-being.*

Recent scientific developments have affirmed and refined Freud's thesis. Evolutionary psychologists have identified sex as the linchpin of the Darwinian struggle of all creatures to reproduce, advance, and evolve. And in the past ten years neuroscience and psychopharmacology have illuminated another intriguing dimension of our sexuality: Sex is not a stand-alone, "closed" system; rather, it's intricately woven into the web of our bodily systems. When our bodies are in balance—when the digestive, endocrine, circulatory, and other vital systems are functioning at full capacity—our sexual system reflects that state of health and vitality. But, if medications, diet, or other factors have thrown our bodies out of balance, our sexuality may well become the innocent bystander caught in the crossfire.

I've kept sex for the last chapter of this book because all the other components of the Antidepressant Survival Program—good nutrition, exercise, relaxation and play and spirituality, hormonal and digestive health—are building blocks of healthy sexuality.

And in the same way that sexuality reflects broader physical and psychic health, a healthy sex drive affects much more than sex life. It's the creative, engaging life force that we bring to every aspect of our lives: our work, our friendships, and of course our most intimate relationships. That is why sexual dysfunction should never be dismissed— by either you or your doctor—as a necessary "cost" of escaping the grasp of depression. Healthy sexuality is a critical key to reclaiming a fulfilling and engaged life. Our abilities to connect with others and to achieve intimacy are nature's antidotes to the isolation depression leaves in its wake. And our feelings of desirability and empowerment are crucial to our ability to express our creativity and navigate success-fully in the world.

A twenty-five-year-old patient of mine named Maxine told me that having sex on Prozac felt like a visit to the gynecologist. "I miss the sen-sation, the sexual pleasures and the release, but I also miss the feeling of power," she said, "that feeling of excitement I get when I can enter a room and turn a few heads. That power is gone because I no longer feel sexy."

You, too, may feel like someone has pulled the plug on your sex life. You may not enjoy sex, or you may even find it's uncomfortable. You may have forgotten what it is like to feel desirable, sexy. Whatever problems you're experiencing, you need to recognize the fact that anti-depressants—or several other factors I'll highlight—could be the cul-prits. You may be experiencing one or a number of these symptoms as a result of taking antidepressants.

YOUR SEXUAL FUNCTIONING

The sexual side effects caused by antidepressants have become more well known in recent years. Some drugs, like Prozac, were approved by the Food and Drug Administration without any indication that they

Sexual Self-Evaluation

1. Has your interest in or desire for sex been decreased before or since you began taking antidepressants?

2. Men, do you have difficulty maintaining an erection?

3. Do you have a sense of numbness or reduced sensitivity in your genital area when touched?

4. Do you find that you rarely or never achieve orgasm or that it takes more time to achieve?

5. Men, do you have difficulty with penetration? Women, do you find intercourse painful because you've had a change in lubrication during sex?

6. Is your intimate relationship, or willingness to get involved in a relationship, being affected by any sexual problems?

7. Do you feel unconcerned about your lack of a sex life?

If you answered yes to any of these questions, you may be experiencing a side effect of antidepressants or be suffering from an undiagnosed problem that affects your sexuality.

---

caused significant sexual problems. In clinical trials conducted to receive FDA approval, the manufacturers of Prozac found that only 1.6 percent of patients experienced decreased libido and only 1.9 percent experienced sexual dysfunction. Soon after Prozac was approved in 1988, however, psychiatrists began to find that sexual side effects were much more common, so researchers started to study the problem. One study found that 62 percent of people who take Prozac or some other SSRI can't achieve orgasm, and 75 percent of men have trouble maintaining an erection. (In fact, these medications are now being prescribed to men who have premature ejaculation because they are so effective at delaying orgasm.)

As a student of the brain, I have not been surprised to learn that normal sexual functioning is the result of a tightly connected, symphonic coordination of these chemical systems and hormones with one's psychological and social environment. A significant disturbance in any aspect of this symphony will disturb your sexuality—and in the long run your general well-being and health—to a greater or lesser degree.

The most recent research on how antidepressants affect sexual functioning points to the action of these medications on certain chemical systems in the brain and spinal cord—neurotransmitters and receptors. It is clear that different antidepressants affect different combinations of these neurotransmitters and receptors, causing one or more sexual problems: decreased desire for sex, decreased sensation and pleasure, decreased erection or vaginal wetness, and difficulty having an orgasm or full climax.

If you've suffered the debilitating effects of depression or some other medical condition, you may have forgotten what it's like to have good, satisfying sex. In fact, some of my patients don't notice much of a change in their sex lives after going on antidepressants because their sexual desires have been buried for so long. Frequently, it will be your spouse or partner who brings the problem to your attention.

Please take my advice and listen to your loved one. Your mind-body pathways can't function optimally without sexual vitality, nor can your love relationship. A growing body of research indicates that those who have an active, satisfying sex life have improved health and longevity. Obviously, the benefits of sex extend beyond the bedroom to your mind, body, and spirit. Do not let antidepressants rob you of this vital life force. Work the Antidepressant Survival Program fully and you will reclaim it.

A FOUR-STEP APPROACH TO RECLAIMING YOUR SEXUAL VITALITY

The good news is that we now know much more about how antidepressants cause sexual dysfunction. And, as you've no doubt heard, there are now readily available drugs that can restore full sexual function for most people. Beyond Viagra, and its sibling medications now coming onto the market, there are other strategies that work for reclaiming a healthy and vital sex life.

You may have skipped straight from the table of contents to this chapter, looking for a quick fix for your problem. That's human nature—but *starting with this chapter isn't necessarily the shortest path to a solution.* Many of my patients find that simply following the Fundamentals of good nutrition, exercise, and stress reduction has a therapeutic effect on their sex lives. As I point out in the earlier chapters, good eating habits and increased circulation from exercise, along with improved self-esteem and sense of physical desirability, are important components of sexual vitality. And correcting the hormonal problems discussed in Chapter 8 often also has a very significant, positive impact on desire and performance.

I've developed a four-step program to help you reclaim your sexual vitality.

1. Assess your sexual hormone levels and see if you need any supplementation.
2. Evaluate the impact of your antidepressant on your sexuality and consider changing or adjusting your medication.
3. Use herbal therapies.
4. Use sexual enhancers, such as Viagra and other medications.

One or all of these steps should prove useful to you. I recommend that you begin with Step 1 and continue through the program until you're happy with the results. You'll need to follow this program under your doctor's supervision—which means you'll have to have a frank discussion with your doctor about your sex life. This can be a surprisingly difficult first step, but I urge you not to shy away from it.

Perhaps you can start by writing the problem out on paper, then discussing it with a friend, your spouse, or your therapist. Give serious consideration to having your therapist clear the path with your doctor ahead of time in a letter or by phone. Then schedule an extralong session with your doctor so that neither of you feels rushed. Prepare what you want to say in writing, so that you are sure you cover your major feelings and problems. Or you can give your doctor a copy of this book or this chapter as an icebreaker. However you decide to go about it, please allow your doctor to become your partner in treating this medical problem. I can assure you that it is too important to your mind-body health to ignore.

If, having done all these things to alert him or her to the special concerns you have, your doctor dismisses your sexual side effects as a minor problem, or as "better than being depressed," find yourself a new doctor.

NINE FACTORS (BESIDES ANTIDEPRESSANTS) THAT WREAK HAVOC ON YOUR SEX LIFE

Before you assume that antidepressants are the cause of your sexual problems, ask yourself the following questions to see whether another factor may be involved. Review this list with your doctor.

1. Are you aroused by others but not your partner?

If so, you may need to work on your relationship.

2. Do you still feel depressed at times?

If your depression is not fully alleviated, you could have a low sex drive. Or you may have a low estrogen or testosterone level, which can mimic depression and prevent your antidepressant from working fully.

3. Do you have coronary artery disease or high levels of cholesterol?

If you have narrowed arteries, you may have reduced blood flow to your sex organs, which could cause erection problems or prevent orgasm. Consult your doctor about changing your diet and lifestyle (in concert with the other parts of the program) and about whether you need medications to lower your cholesterol or blood pressure.

4. Do you have diabetes?

This condition, in which the body is unable to regulate blood-sugar levels, frequently causes sexual problems by damaging nerves and reducing blood flow to sex organs. If you have any of the symptoms of diabetes (frequent urination, excessive thirst, weight gain, sugar cravings, slow wound healing) as well as sexual dysfunction, you should get a blood test to check for the condition. Your doctor may be able to prescribe a medication like Viagra to increase blood flow.

5. Do you have an enlarged prostate?

Men with enlarged prostates frequently have trouble maintaining an erection and initiating or maintaining urine flow. If you are a man over age fifty, have your prostate gland evaluated by your doctor.

6. Do you smoke?

Research has shown that 66 percent of male smokers have problems maintaining an erection. Female smokers may have problems experiencing pleasure and orgasm. The nicotine in cigarettes causes your blood vessels to constrict, and the various chemicals in the cigarette smoke cause a buildup of plaque in your arteries, both of which reduce blood flow to your sex organs. The good news is that once you quit smoking these side effects will reverse themselves.

7. Do you drink?

Alcohol, while it reduces inhibitions initially, is a depressant of both sexual function and mood. That nightly glass of red wine with dinner—which can be good for the heart—can be the source of your sexual dysfunction as well.

8. Are you taking any prescription medications besides antidepressants?

A host of medications can lower your sex drive, raise your threshold for orgasm, or cause erection difficulties. Common offenders include antihistamines, stomach acid blockers, antipsychotics, tranquilizers, blood pressure medications, and heart medications. Ask your doctor if your other medications could be interfering with your sex life.

9. Do you do a lot of road biking?

There is evidence that prolonged sitting on a bicycle seat can injure the blood vessels leading to and from the genitals, causing impotence problems for men. Make sure you stand off the seat frequently while biking or switch to a donut-shaped seat, now available for most bikes.

In all of these situations, antidepressants may still play a role in your sexual problems, but you should consult your doctor to sort out the causes and which treatments would work best for you.

STEP ONE:
GETTING YOUR SEX HORMONES ASSESSED

If you've found that your sex drive is low, you may have low levels of certain sex hormones. In Chapter 8 I mentioned that when your body is stressed by illness, your adrenal glands go into overdrive and pump out large amounts of cortisol. If this stress goes on for a while, the adrenal glands get stingy with their production of the sex hormone precursor DHEA. Your body is sending you a clear message: Don't think about sex when you're fighting just to survive.

With less DHEA, your body can't manufacture normal amounts of testosterone and estrogen, the hormones that fuel your sexual desires. As a result, you lose interest in having sex. The trouble is, once your illness is treated, your adrenals don't always get the message that your survival is no longer threatened. For a variety of reasons (such as incompletely treated depression, poor diet, zinc deficiency, high stress levels, and intermittent feelings of helplessness), your DHEA or testosterone levels may remain low.

Part of the reason could be aging. As you approach your forties, your body naturally starts to produce less testosterone. For a woman, this reduction happens along with a decline in estrogen and progesterone as her body prepares for menopause. For a man, testosterone levels drop as he experiences what some researchers refer to as male menopause. Low testosterone levels can also be caused by physical stress (you've embarked on an exercise program that's too strenuous or you're in pain from a medical condition) or emotional stress, which triggers your adrenal glands to slow production of DHEA.

Several pieces of research have found that low testosterone levels frequently cause symptoms that mimic depression, such as depressed moods, irritability, and fatigue. A significant number of my patients have told me that their antidepressants aren't working when they actually have low testosterone levels. Andrew, a thirty-five-year-old advertising copywriter, was one such case. He had been suffering from severe depression, and his doctor prescribed Serzone. After taking the medication for a few months, he felt a little better but found that he still had feelings of deep despair whenever he missed a deadline or got mixed reviews on a project at work. What drove Andrew to see me, though, was the fact that he no longer had any interest in meeting women or having sex. "The other night an attractive woman I met at a party asked for my phone number," he said. "I lied. I told her I was seeing someone and just walked away."

I knew Andrew probably wasn't experiencing a side effect from his antidepressant, since Serzone rarely causes sexual problems. So I decided to run a blood test to check his free testosterone. The level was half as high as it should have been for his age, so I prescribed a testosterone cream, which I told Andrew to apply to his scrotum every morning and noon. Several weeks later he told me that he had been out on a few dates and that his old sexual urges had begun to reawaken. He said that he now felt only mild disappointment over things that usually caused him despair; his antidepressant was working much better. He also noted that he felt mentally sharper than he had in several years.

If you are experiencing any sexual problems, I recommend you have a blood test to determine your testosterone levels. Your doctor should obtain a measure of free testosterone, the active component of the hormone that circulates in your bloodstream to boost sex drive. If your testosterone levels are low, after a thorough workup your doctor will probably prescribe a testosterone supplement in the form of a cream, patch, or pills. I find that the cream usually works best and is reportedly the least likely to cause liver damage—a rare but serious side effect of testosterone supplementation. More common side effects of testosterone supplements are bloating, acne, hair thinning, shrinkage of the testicles, and temporary enlargement of breast tissue (in both men and women). You should not be given testosterone if you have had breast cancer (men or women) or prostate cancer.

NOTE TO YOUR DOCTOR

Assessing Testosterone Production

A thorough blood workup should include measuring free testosterone. (I also recommend a measure of serum prolactin, hemoglobin A_1C, and thyroid hormones to rule out other medical conditions.) If testosterone levels are low, I recommend testing zinc, DHEA, luteinizing hormone, and follicle-stimulating hormone to determine the exact nature of the problem. If any of these levels are low or low-normal, a repeat assay should be done for confirmation, since there is a wide variability in the accuracy of the various laboratory kits. Normal ranges also vary from lab to lab, so your patient's symptoms should be correlated with the medical history and any past history of substance abuse in addition to the lab findings.

If your patient's level of testosterone falls below the percentile of the normal age-adjusted range and the zinc is normal, you should consider testosterone supplementation. For male patients, I prefer a topical cream (obtainable at compounding pharmacies such as the Apothecary, 301-530-0800), applied to the scrotum in the morning and at noon; the cream eliminates the fluctuations in mood, sex drive, and energy that can occur with the injectable form, which is administered every two to four weeks (for example, testosterone cypionate 200 to 400 milligrams). Also, the cream is unlikely to cause liver disturbances. I start with a 10 percent testosterone cream (which eliminates the irritation often caused by patches), having the patient apply

.50 gram in the morning and .25 gram at noon. After two to four weeks I measure the patient's free testosterone level (trough and peak) and note any changes in symptoms. I then adjust the dosage accordingly. Possible side effects from testosterone include an increase in the hematocrit, increased platelet aggregation, temporary enlargement of breast tissue, water retention, acne, hair loss, reduction in the size of the testicles, and worsening of sleep apnea.

When prescribing testosterone, liver and prostate function must be monitored via physical exam, complete blood cell count, liver function tests, and free PSA. Although no association has been found between the administration of testosterone and prostate cancer, it is known that male hormones (androgens) can stimulate the growth of already diagnosed prostate cancer; moreover, benign prostatic hypertrophy can become more severe with testosterone supplementation.

If your patient is female, you may also want to consider testosterone supplementation, especially if she is menopausal. I've found that the cream (applied to the labia at one-third the male dose—a 3.5 percent cream) generally works the best. Such supplementation must be done carefully and under close supervision, since excessive dosages can cause virilization, which may not be reversible. A micronized oral capsule can be started at morning and lunch if your patient does not prefer to use a cream, beginning with 2.5 milligrams at each dose.

STEP TWO:
CONSIDER SWITCHING ANTIDEPRESSANTS OR ALTERING THEIR TIMING

Martin, a thirty-three-year-old father of two, knew he needed to take antidepressants for the rest of his life to keep him from crashing into another severe depression, like the one that had left him dangerously suicidal two years before. Taking a combination of three antidepressants—lithium, Prozac, and Pamelor—that I prescribed, Martin was able to resume running his own business and enjoying his sons' Little

League games. Still, an important part of his life was missing: He had no desire for sex. "My wife and I haven't had sex since I started my medications," Martin told me. "But I don't really feel like I miss it."

Martin and his wife, Sue, came to me to discuss this aspect of Martin's life. As it turned out, Martin had a reduced sex drive as well as decreased sensation and difficulty with orgasm. I explained to Martin and Sue that all three of his antidepressants were known to have a negative impact on sexual function. We decided to slowly replace his Pamelor with the antidepressant Wellbutrin, which is rarely associated with sexual problems and is actually helpful for these problems. Martin later reported to me that within days of adding the Wellbutrin he felt like a teenager again. He told me he had fantasized about having sex with his wife on his desk at work. "I called my wife and told her about my fantasy," he recalled with a broad grin. "When I got home, the kids were at my mother's and we had sex on the desk in our study." (I'd call that a successful treatment outcome.)

The neurochemicals involved in sexual functions are serotonin, adrenaline, acetylcholine, dopamine, and nitric oxide. While the subtypes of sexual problems you may experience (decreased desire, sensation, and so on) are fairly distinct, the effects of antidepressants on these aspects of your sexuality are more muddled. Thus, a so-called purely serotonergic antidepressant, such as Prozac, actually has secondary effects on dopamine, while the very highly selective serotonergic antidepressant Paxil has secondary effects on acetylcholine. This means that you are probably experiencing more than one sexual dysfunction at a time; you may have decreased desire as well as trouble with climax, or you may have decreased lubrication as well as diminished sensation but still be able to climax with effort.

The incidence of sexual side effects varies from medication to medication, but the SSRI inhibitors—early on hailed as side effect free—are among the worst offenders. In his recent review, entitled "The role of antidepressants in sexual dysfunction" (*Journal of Clinical Psychiatry,* monograph 17, no. 1, March 1999: 9–14), Dr. Norman Sussman confirms my clinical impression that the incidence of sexual dysfunction is between 50 and 70 percent.

It is clear that all the SSRIs (and the older antidepressants as well) cause sexual dysfunction; however, there are some differences that you should consider in light of your sexual problem. Paxil, the most potent serotonergic agent among the SSRIs, is the most likely to cause sexual dysfunction. In particular, complete inability to achieve orgasm or ejaculation, as well as impotence, was most frequently associated with Paxil. There was no difference among the SSRIs for severity of decreased libido and delayed (not inhibited) orgasm or ejaculation.

There are six antidepressants currently on the market that rarely or never cause sexual side effects: Wellbutrin, Remeron, Serzone, Deseryl, St. John's wort, and SAM-e. Wellbutrin has a different mechanism of action than the serotonin reuptake inhibitors. Serzone and Remeron actually block the serotonin from binding to the 5-HT_2 receptor (which seems to be responsible for the sexual side effects of serotonin antidepressants). One study found that more than 80 percent of people with sexual problems who switched from an SSRI to Wellbutrin experienced an improvement in their libido, orgasms, and overall sexual satisfaction. SAM-e is a new substance available in health-food stores that early studies have shown to be helpful (especially when used intravenuously for depression) without sexual side effects. However, the same caveats about purity I've noted about St. John's wort apply to this substance. A therapeutic dose of SAM-e is typically 300 to 400 milligrams three times a day.

It's worth it to try switching medications as long as your doctor keeps close track of your symptoms to make sure that your depression does not recur. If the medication you are using is working well to alleviate your depression, it may be possible, under your doctor's supervision, to add small doses of these medications (Wellbutrin, Remeron, Serzone) to your regimen. For example, Milt, a forty-two-year-old attorney I was treating, found that Prozac had alleviated his depression, panic attacks, and obsessive-compulsive disorder. However, his libido was lower and he had less sensation during sex and was unable to maintain an erection. I added a very, very small dose (10 milligrams) of Serzone to his regimen, and his sex drive and function returned. (Adding Serzone to an SSRI must be done very cautiously because of possible drug interactions.)

As with any medication, these three antidepressants have some side effects and caveats. Wellbutrin SR (slow release) can be a bit inconvenient to take, since doses must be carefully timed ten to twelve hours apart. Wellbutrin also can have a slightly higher risk of causing seizures under certain conditions and should not be taken if you have ever had a seizure, significant head trauma, anorexia or bulimia, or if you are taking a monoamine oxidase (MAO) inhibitor. I also advise my patients to avoid caffeine and alcohol completely because these can theoretically combine with the medication to raise the risk of seizures.

Remeron's most troublesome side effect is weight gain. I've seen patients gain upwards of ten pounds on the drug because of increased cravings for sweets. The best way to battle this side effect is to follow the Fundamentals. Serzone, which is relatively new, can cause sedation, so your dose must be increased gradually to find the most effective dose with the fewest side effects.

Desyrel, an antidepressant with few sexual side effects, is not an option for men since it can cause prolonged and painful erections. In women, however, it works extremely well to increase arousal during sex and make it easier to achieve orgasm. Desyrel can be added in small doses to your medication regimen (although you can't take it if you are on an MAO inhibitor).

Note: Switching antidepressants may not be an option for some patients whose depression or medical condition requires a combination of antidepressants. I should also note that switching from one SSRI to another—for example, Prozac to Luvox or Zoloft—can work for some people. It is not clear exactly why, but for some people one SSRI causes severe sexual problems while another has no such effect.

If you cannot switch your medications, try altering the timing of your dose. The goal is to have the lowest concentration of antidepressant in your bloodstream around the time you normally have sex. This requires a little advance planning and may take some of the spontaneity out of sex, but I've found that it works surprisingly well for some patients, like a twenty-six-year-old patient of mine named Megan. Megan had been taking Paxil for depression and obsessive-compulsive disorder for six months. During one visit she told me that she and her boyfriend, Rick, were on the outs. "I feel so isolated from him," she said. "We never seem to connect anymore." As I questioned Megan further, I found out that she and her boyfriend had not had sex in four months. "At first, we just cuddled, but I would stop him before we had intercourse. Now that Rick knows it's not going to go any further, he's stopped touching me altogether," she said.

It turned out that sex had changed for Megan soon after she started taking the Paxil. She told me that intercourse had become painful because she had less lubrication. She also stopped having orgasms. "Rick can't seem to understand why I don't want to do something that gives me no pleasure and causes me pain," she said with annoyance.

Megan and I discussed her options. Since her depression and obsessive-compulsive disorder were being well managed by the Paxil, we decided not to reduce her dose. I told her about my program and suggested specific ways to improve her diet. We also designed an exercise plan Megan could commit to. On her next visit, one month later, Megan said she felt an increase in energy, felt better about her body, and noticed that on a few occasions she had a desire to have sex. She and Rick had one encounter, but she said she didn't feel much pleasure and couldn't get close to orgasm.

"When do you usually take your evening dose of medication, and what time did you have sex that night?" I asked. Megan told me she regularly took the Paxil at 7:00 P.M. with dinner, and that she and Rick used to have sex around 10:00 P.M. The night they had sex, she happened to miss her 7:00 P.M. dose. I knew Megan needed a more complete solution and thought it might lie in timing.

"Your problem may be that you have the highest concentration of the drug in your bloodstream at the time you have sex," I explained. I told Megan to try taking the antidepressant after sex and just before bedtime, rather than with dinner. I also encouraged her to increase her exercise further. On her next visit Megan told me that her sex life was back in full swing. She began having regular orgasms during her sexual encounters and, using a lubricant gel, no longer felt pain during intercourse. She told me she couldn't believe that the solution to her problem was so simple.

If you decide to alter the timing of your dose, the simplest rule of thumb is to take it after having sex. It's better to take your medication at the same time every day, so you don't forget to take a dose. If you usually have sex at 10:00 P.M., for example, take your last dose

around 11:00 each night. If you tend to have sex first thing in the morning, take a pill an hour after you would normally have sex and take
your second dose (if you usually take two doses) in the early or
midafternoon.

Note: Some doctors favor reducing the dose of antidepressant to alleviate sexual side effects, but I don't recommend this because it puts you
at risk for a recurrence of your depression. A very significant amount
of research has found that the dose that gets you well keeps you well.
Unless you were quickly put on a high dosage of antidepressant (without being given gradual increases to your current dose), it is unlikely
that your dosage is too high.

NOTE TO YOUR DOCTOR

Managing Sexual Dysfunction

The importance of an active, satisfying sex life in the maintenance of health, mental and physical, cannot be ignored.
Isolation, as a result of a diminished or absent sex life, contributes
to relapse or recurrence of depression. Once the depression has
been treated, I suggest that the sexual side effects of the antidepressants be explored and given appropriate priority. According
to recent research, failure to do so has numerous health consequences (including decreased longevity) and increases the risk of
noncompliance with the medication and subsequent recurrence
of the presenting symptoms. Studies by Dr. Robert Post indicate
that each depressive episode results in increased sensitivity to a
depressive occurrence: Depression begets depression, and thus it
is incumbent upon us to address those problems, such as sexual
difficulties, that affect compliance.

Changing medications is a viable alternative in patients whose
depressions are readily responsive to medication, but in patients
who have struggled to find an effective regimen, this may not be
advisable. In these cases I recommend you support and encourage your patient to follow the entire program outlined in this
book, as well as use the interventions in this chapter.

STEP THREE:
TAKING HERBAL SUPPLEMENTS

Certain herbal supplements can be a useful option in many cases of sexual dysfunction. One word of caution: Herbs used as drugs or pharmaceuticals (often called herbaceuticals) are not benign and generally have as much potential for side effects and harm as medications that are prescribed by your doctor, since they are combinations of biologically active chemicals. Another problem is that herbs are not regulated for quality control as drugs are, so you need to be careful to buy brands that are of high quality. (You can ask your pharmacist for recommended brands.) Herbal products should have the word "standardized" on their labels, which means that the manufacturer tries to get the same potency of herb in every pill.

Ginkgo biloba, which comes from an ancient tree, has been shown in early studies, and in my patients, to increase libido and help achieve orgasm and maintain an erection. Ginkgo may increase blood flow by making blood vessels more flexible and red blood cells more pliable, so cells can squeeze through tiny capillaries without getting stuck. Perhaps this enables blood to reach the genitals (and the other primary sex organ, the brain). More research is needed to support these claims, but one study found that ginkgo increased desire, arousal, and orgasm in men and women who had sexual problems as a result of taking antidepressants. Another study found that the herb could increase sensation in the sex organs. Other studies have contradicted these results, but ginkgo works in enough of my patients that I consider it a very reasonable intervention. Ginkgo has additional beneficial effects on memory and, according to several studies, helps protect nerve cells from oxidant damage.

I recommend the Nature's Way brand of ginkgo called Ginkgold because it is produced by the same company that produced the ginkgo for the numerous clinical trials in Germany. It contains high-quality ginkgo, while other products may not. Start by taking one 60-milligram tablet every day. After one week increase to two tablets per day. Work your way up to six tablets per day over six weeks, if necessary. Allow two to three months to determine whether the ginkgo has helped you. Cut back on your dose if you experience any side effects,

such as nausea, restlessness, diarrhea, or vomiting. Use gingko with caution if you take aspirin regularly or an anticoagulant medication, or you have a condition in which bleeding would be dangerous (for example, stomach ulcer).

Ginseng is another herb that I recommend to patients. It comes in two forms: Panax and Siberian. The herb contains chemicals called gensenosides (also called panaxosides), which are thought to improve sexual functioning. Panax ginseng is considered more potent and may be useful if you lack energy and want to increase your libido and pleasure. Some reports indicate that Panax can make erections more rigid and longer lasting, although there is little firm data to support these claims. Ginseng is expensive (selling for as much as twenty to thirty dollars per ounce in Asian markets) and can be purchased in health-food stores as a tonic, powder, or capsule. Follow the instructions on the package for dosing. Side effects can include insomnia, high blood pressure, diarrhea, restlessness, anxiety, and euphoria. Ginseng should not be taken if you are on an MAO inhibitor, since it can make this antidepressant dangerously potent.

Yohimbine is a potent herb made from the pulverized bark of the African tree yohimbé. It is thought to boost sex drive and improve sexual function. Until Viagra came onto the market, yohimbine was the only FDA-approved pill for the treatment of impotence. One meta-analysis of seven studies found that men with erectile dysfunction who took yohimbine were nearly four times as likely to have successful intercourse as men who took a placebo. Yohimbine is available in health-food stores, but I don't recommend using an over-the-counter preparation since a 1995 analysis of twenty-six commercial yohimbine products found that most contain little or virtually no yohimbine. Instead, you should use the prescription Yocon (yohimbine) under your doctor's supervision. Side effects can occur and include anxiety, nervousness, palpitations, and panic attacks. These side effects are even more likely if you are taking an MAO inhibitor or a tricyclic antidepressant.

St. John's wort, an herbal antidepressant, is associated with fewer sexual side effects than the SSRIs. It is useful in mild to moderate depressions, according to a metaanalysis of several studies recently published in the *British Journal of Medicine*. St. John's wort seems to take

four to six weeks to work. Recently, a pharmaceutical grade brand of St. John's wort called Alterra was released by a major pharmaceutical company. Its appeal is the notion that this brand will have better quality control than the over-the-counter brands. I recommend that you use either Kira brand St. John's wort (available in health-food stores without a prescription) or Alterra.

St. John's wort should not be combined with other antidepressants because its exact mechanism of action is not known but may include MAO inhibition. If that is a significant mode of action, then mixing St. John's wort with other antidepressants could lead to severe, and even life-threatening, elevations of blood pressure.

STEP FOUR:
CONSIDER TAKING VIAGRA—
EVEN IF YOU'RE A WOMAN

"Viagra has become to erectile dysfunction what Prozac was for depression," says the psychiatrist Troy Thompson, a colleague of mine who spoke at a recent American Psychiatric Association meeting in Toronto. Since coming onto the market in March 1998, Viagra has had a dramatic effect on the way doctors treat the sexual side effects caused by antidepressants. Suddenly men who were not able to maintain an erection could be treated with a pill—rather than cumbersome penile pumps or (ouch!) injectable drugs. The press quickly dubbed Viagra "a wonder drug, a modern aphrodisiac" and likened it to the Pill for women. Another medication, called Vasomax, should be approved by the FDA by 2000 and works similarly to Viagra.

As is often the case in science, Viagra came about by accident. Researchers at Pfizer were trying to invent a chest pain medication for heart disease patients. Viagra was supposed to reduce chest pain by increasing blood flow through the heart. It failed to do this, but it did increase blood flow to the penis, resulting in erections in the volunteers who took it. Viagra works by boosting one aspect of the chemical process that creates an erection. When an erection occurs, a chemical called cyclic GMP binds to muscle cells in the erectile tissue of the penis (and perhaps clitoris), which causes the cells to manufacture nitric oxide. When nitric oxide is released from the cells, it relaxes arteries in the penis and allows blood to flow in, causing an erection. Viagra blocks the effects of an enzyme called phosphodiesterase type 5, which normally breaks down cyclic GMP before it can bind to cells. The drug works so specifically on this process that it does not usually cause increased blood flow to other areas of the body, which could result in unwanted side effects.

One study published in *The New England Journal of Medicine* of 532 men with erectile dysfunction found that men who took Viagra were able to have intercourse 69 percent of the time, compared with 22 percent of the time in the men who took a placebo. Other studies have found that Viagra can improve the quality of sex and boost sex drive. I've found that Viagra has brought new hope to men who have had little success with other options.

Tom, a forty-year-old electrical engineer, had always had an active sex life and took a certain pride in his sexual exploits. Previously married and divorced, Tom was now content to have a series of relatively brief relationships. He and one particular girlfriend enjoyed having sex in the woods and open fields when they went camping. For the past few months, though, Tom had become extremely self-conscious about sex. He had been taking the antidepressant Paxil for depression and anxiety attacks. The medication was working, but Tom was having difficulty maintaining an erection. "The other night, I watched my girlfriend take her clothes off in a really sexy way, peeling them off piece by piece. I got a hard-on, but then my erection vanished as quickly as it started," he told me. "She gave me oral sex, but it took me ten minutes to climax and we couldn't have intercourse." When Viagra came onto the market, Tom called me immediately, and I prescribed the medication. He found that it completely cleared up the sexual side effects from the Paxil. "I don't worry anymore about whether I'll be able to perform during sex," he said.

What about Viagra for women?

That's what one woman asked her doctor. Joanne, a thirty-seven-year-old mother of two, was depressed after she had a hysterectomy for uterine cancer. She began to experience extreme anxiety and felt as if her world had collapsed around her. She was even contemplating suicide. Her gynecologist prescribed Prozac to relieve her depression, and

Joanne's moods improved. But she noticed a troubling side effect: Sex with her husband, which had not been that pleasurable since the hysterectomy, had become a nonevent. "I feel completely numb whenever my husband enters me," she told her doctor. "I may as well be asleep." Joanne had heard that some researchers were testing Viagra in women, and she wondered if the drug could work for her.

Joanne's doctor referred her to some colleagues of mine at the Women's Sexual Health Clinic at the Boston University School of Medicine. They enrolled her in a research study and gave her a prescription for Viagra, instructing her to take it about an hour before she had sex. After taking the pill, Joanne noticed a dramatic improvement. She experienced a resurgence of sexual pleasure and with some tender stroking from her husband was able to have an orgasm. Joanne remained on the Prozac and continues to use Viagra to enhance her sex life.

Since Viagra was approved only for use in men (which means that women were not included in the manufacturer's clinical trials), doctors still don't know whether the drug can increase a woman's sex drive or allow her to experience more pleasure during sex. The few small studies that have been published have reached conflicting conclusions. One study, from Columbia University Medical School, of thirty-three postmenopausal women who were put on Viagra for sexual dysfunction (lack of orgasm, lubrication, clitoral sensation) found that only 18 percent of patients had a significant therapeutic response. Researchers from the Massachusetts General Hospital in Boston came to a much more hopeful conclusion: Viagra was found to improve significantly the sexual satisfaction (libido, arousal, orgasm) of nine men and five women who had sexual problems as a result of taking an SSRI inhibitor. Sixty-nine percent of participants reported significant improvement in their sexual satisfaction (libido, arousal, orgasm) after taking Viagra. What's more, the researchers found that the women had the same degree of improvement as the men.

Scientists have also conducted an experiment to see if Viagra can induce "an erection" in a woman's clitoris. Researchers from Boston University School of Medicine studied Viagra's effects on clitoral muscle tissue samples that were grown in petri dishes. They found that clitoral muscle tissue contains the enzyme phosphodiesterase type 5 and that Viagra inhibits this enzyme. The researchers concluded that Viagra appears to boost the chemical pathways that enable the clitoris to fill with blood and allow a woman to have an orgasm.

I have recently begun to prescribe Viagra to women, and I monitor them on follow-up visits to see whether the medication is working for them. I think Viagra may be a good option to try if you haven't found a solution to your sexual problems. Remember, you don't need to make a long-term commitment. You can try the pill once or twice to see whether it works for you.

Viagra, like any medication, has some side effects that you should be aware of. These include headache, flushing, stomach upset, and temporary visual disturbances, such as increased sensitivity to light, blurred vision, or color tinge. Also, Viagra should not be taken if you are on blood pressure medication that contains organic nitrates (for example, Nitro-Dur).

If your doctor rules out Viagra for you, other medications may be an option. If you are taking an SSRI inhibitor, a drug called amantadine can help increase sexual pleasure and orgasm. Ritalin has been useful in some patients. If you are taking one of the tricyclic antidepressants (Pamelor, Elavil, Norpramin), a medication called bethanechol can help reverse the inhibition of orgasm that commonly occurs with these antidepressants.

NOTE TO YOUR DOCTOR

Medicating Sexual Side Effects

There are numerous medications that can be used to enhance the various sexual dysfunctions accompanying the use of antidepressant medications. The following chart can be used as a guide. Try one medication from each category, for instance, a dopamine agonist (amantadine, bupropion, or methylphenidate), a cholinomimetic (for example, bethanechol), a serotonin blocker (for example, cyproheptadine), or an alpha agonist (for example, Yocon). Observe for effects. If it is beneficial but causes some side effects, try another medication in the same category. If it has no effect, try a different category that relates to the pharmacology of the drug and the pathophysiology of the dysfunction.

Group	Clinical Use
Dopaminergic/ noradrenergic medications	This group of medications generally increases pleasure and sexual desire, as well as orgasm, erection, and vaginal lubrication.
Wellbutrin (bupropion)	Used often as a sole agent in the treatment of depression (as it is free of sexual effects), but also very effective to augment efficacy of serotonergic antidepressants and alleviate decreased desire, pleasure, and orgasm (use in smaller doses). May be used daily, or as needed 1–2 hours before sexual activity.
Ritalin (methylphenidate)	Very effective to augment efficacy of serotonergic antidepressants and alleviate decreased desire, pleasure, and orgasm caused by serotonergic antidepressants.
Symmetrel (amantadine)	Reported to be effective to augment efficacy of serotonergic antidepressants and alleviate decreased desire, pleasure, and orgasm caused by serotonergic antidepressants.
Dexedrine (dextroamphetamine)	Very effective to augment efficacy of serotonergic antidepressants and alleviate decreased desire, pleasure, and orgasm caused by serotonergic antidepressants.
Yohimbine (Yocon)	This medication—an herb—is very useful in erectile dysfunction in males (and perhaps clitoral erectile dysfunction in females) and can be taken on an as-needed basis 1–2 hours before intercourse.

(continued on next page)

Group	Clinical Use
Vasomax (phentolamine mesylate)	Phase-three clinical studies have been completed; should be released soon. Useful in erectile dysfunction in males (and perhaps clitoral erectile dysfunction in females) and can be taken on an as-needed basis 1–2 hours before intercourse.
Serotonin blockers (antagonists)	This group of medications blocks the activity of serotonin at specific receptors. They can be useful in attenuating the decreased sensation, difficulty with orgasm, and perhaps the decreased desire that accompany the serotonergic antidepressants. They may cause temporary relapse of depressive or other symptomatology in some people.
Periactin (cyproheptadine)	Taken about 2 hours before sexual activity.
Serzone (nefazodone)	Used in low dosages, taken daily; may be carefully added to many antidepressants. Reportedly effective in attenuating the decreased sensation, difficulty with orgasm, and decreased desire that accompany the serotonergic antidepressants.
Remeron (mirtazapine)	Reported in some cases to be useful in attenuating the decreased sensation, difficulty with orgasm, and perhaps decreased desire that accompany the serotonergic antidepressants.

Group	Clinical Use
Buspar (buspirone)	In higher doses (over 30 mg) has been reported to be useful in attenuating the decreased sensation, difficulty with orgasm, and perhaps decreased desire that accompany the serotonergic antidepressants.
Cholinergic medications	This group is primarily useful with tricyclics, which have strong anticholinergic effects, as well as for the occasional person who experiences anticholinergic effects from other medications (e.g., Effexor, Paxil).
Bethanechol (urecholine)	Helpful in reversing difficulties caused by tricyclics, such as impaired erection and vaginal lubrication. Can be taken on an as-needed basis 1–2 hours before sexual activity. Several trials may be needed to establish effective dose.
Herbals	Herbals have a variety of proposed mechanisms of action. Careful brand selection is necessary.
Ginkgo biloba	Very useful in high doses (about 300 mg of the standardized extract) on a daily basis. Allow 6 weeks for benefit. Useful in improving desire, erection, and orgasm.
Panax ginseng	Use on an as-needed basis. Can be useful in increasing erection and sexual desire.

(continued on next page)

Group	Clinical Use
Phosphodiesterase type 5 inhibitors	Early clinical impressions are that this class may be considered as a first choice in cases of erectile dysfunction and vaginal lubrication, with significant but less efficacy than the dopaminergic/noradrenergic agents in the area of pleasure and sensation.
Viagra (sildenafil)	Used as needed 1 hour before sexual activity.

Note: Consult *PDR* or other sources for potential adverse effects and interactions before use.

Conclusion

* * *

I'VE TALKED A LOT throughout this book about taking control of your health by taking responsibility for your lifestyle—the food you eat, the way you exercise, and how you modulate stress. I want to end by urging you to let yourself taste life, explore life, and fight the tendency to seek security and predictability.

One hot day last summer, while biking after work along the Potomac River, I had the sudden inclination to take a detour off the main path. Since I make it a point on these excursions to follow my curiosity, I turned into the new path with a sense of excitement and curiosity, and a touch of apprehension. Where will this lead, and what new things will I experience?

I turned onto a somewhat challenging single-track mountain bike path that meandered unpredictably along the water's edge. I stopped to enjoy the quiet, and the lush and serene vista before riding onward. I was astounded that I had lived in Washington for over fifteen years and had never experienced the river like this before—just biking, exploring. I was even more amazed that this experience was only fifteen minutes from my door all this time! Suddenly, in the midst of these thoughts, I saw a mother duck leading her fifteen or so ducklings into the water as the sun began to set in the distance, with the smallest duckling trailing behind the others. The mother waited until the littlest duckling waded in. The beauty was inspiring. Hopping back onto my bike, I rode the new trail feeling a sense of the invigoration and energy that make life so worth living. I was in heaven.

As I moved through this new trail, I concentrated my attention on the principles of balance, posture, and integrated body movement necessary to keep the bicycle moving across the various obstacles in my path: rocks, logs, and tree roots. I went through my mental checklist of do's and don'ts. Suddenly I was faced with a sharp bend into a narrow, rock-strewn trail, and I tensed up, focusing intently and automatically—not on where I wanted the bike to go but rather on where I didn't want it to go! Of course, the bike and my body followed my eyes, and I lost control of the bike. I went flying through the air over my handlebars, in slow motion, landing in a pile of bushes.

I was quite rattled. I caught my breath, lying there on my back, and began to enjoy this new perspective of the trees. When I stood up, I found a six-inch scrape on my calf. In a strange way, this too was invigorating, because I hadn't scraped a knee since I was a kid! I was playing again! Again I hopped on my bike and finished the trail, wondering what I had done wrong.

I tackled this new path again the next afternoon, this time focused on keeping myself at one with the bike and keeping my eyes on my chosen path, rather than on the obstacles. I relaxed and felt the rhythm. I nailed it. The trail was mine, and I was in heaven again: this time without falling, and with even more pleasure. I had learned my first real lesson of biking: You don't ride the bike; it moves you best when you are relaxed and you move as one unit with the bike, always staying focused on *where you want to go,* not on where you are afraid you will end up!

Ever since that afternoon, biking has become an essential pleasure of my day, the still point in my hectic and frenetic world. The reason it's so peaceful and sweet is that it's the one time of day when I can relax and enjoy my own company.

These are the final thoughts I'd like to leave you with. Trust your body and mind's instinct toward balance and health. Remain focused on your goals—not your obstacles—and they will be yours.

If you've been struggling for years to find some equilibrium in your life, you may well have come to distrust your body and mind, to view them as your adversaries rather than your allies. Now that you've taken the healthful step of committing to this program, relax and let your body and mind do what comes naturally—return to balance and health. Sure, there will be bumps in the road. But with the help of this program, you'll quickly regain your equilibrium. Your inner compass will steer you true, as long as you *remain focused on where you want to go.*

I appreciate the trust you've put in me by embarking on my program. And I hope you'll extend that trust to whichever doctor you've decided to work with. In the final analysis, though, you need to trust yourself—your body, mind, and spirit's innate talent for knowing what's good for you and moving in that direction. Your body and mind and spirit love good food and exercise and play and relief from stress. If your doctor has corrected certain hormonal or other medical imbalances, your body and mind will appreciate the boost and will thrive.

Most of all, we all need love and trust. Move toward taking care of yourself every day, the way that little boy in the story faithfully watered his carrot seed. And, believe me, you'll get a life—the life *you* envision and create, the life you will enjoy.

Afterword

A Note to My Colleagues

If you are reading this, it is likely that you or your patients have already come up against the limited response to and very troublesome side effects of antidepressant medications, such as weight gain, sexual dysfunction, and fatigue. Over the course of my clinical practice, my teaching at Georgetown University Hospital, the writing of my previous book (*Understanding Biological Psychiatry,* Norton, 1996), and my work with colleagues and patients, I have found that *there are effective remedies for most of these side effects.*

In this book I have outlined key aspects of the approach that I have found extremely helpful to well over three hundred of my patients. Some of these solutions deal directly with side effects, while others treat underlying but overlooked conditions prevalent in the population who use antidepressants. The program is based on medical research in a range of disciplines, including endocrinology, functional medicine, psychopharmacology, gastroenterology, immunology, and nutrition. It synthesizes the findings of these disparate specialties into an integrative approach that other doctors can adapt to their own practices.

All of us who practice clinical medicine have felt helpless in the face of a patient's problems. In situations like these, I find that thinking "out of the box" is my best hope of helping. The program detailed in this book grew out of my own work with treatment-resistant cases in my psychiatric practice. I wasn't comfortable telling my patients that I couldn't help them, and I began delving into the research literature in a wide range of specialties outside my own. What I discovered was that antidepressants (and the disorders prevalent in this population) affect patients pan-systemically—that subclinical pathology present in one system can easily cascade into multiple dysfunctions in other systems, eventually presenting as disease or dysfunction. Because the systems affected by depression and antidepressants are integrated, an integrative treatment approach naturally *evolved* from my investigations.

As you know, the practice of medicine is an endless learning curve. I'm deeply dependent on my patients' collaboration and cooperation, and I draw on the experience and wisdom of other physicians in my field and related ones. I hope you will consider using the information herein as an adjunct to the treatment of your patients. As I've said, no book can replace a doctor-patient relationship built on trust and individual care. Every patient has a unique response to antidepressants, and you remain your patient's best source of medical guidance.

This book is not a training manual, nor should it be used by physicians or patients as such. My goal is to provide you, the physician, with a new road map of innovative techniques for maximizing benefits and managing antidepressant side effects—techniques that I have found highly therapeutic. I have included sections specifically addressed to you (Note to Your Doctor) for your review and direction. These notes include diagnostic and treatment protocols as well as journal citations that reference selected medical research on which these approaches are based. In Appendix One, I've listed the laboratories I've found most reliable, and in Appendix Three, additional medical references.

I have been teaching the principles and techniques of my program to physicians and other health professionals since 1991. For more information, go to my Website—www.wholepsych.com—which is continually updated and revised. I invite you to contact me there with feedback, questions, anecdotes, and suggestions. If you are interested in further training in this approach, you may contact me through American Health Educators, at 301-657-4749.

I appreciate your open-minded and pragmatic approach to solving your patients' problems. I'm confident that the information in this book will offer you valuable new treatment options and improved patient outcomes.

Robert J. Hedaya, M.D.
American Society of Clinical Psychopharmacology
Certified, American Board of Psychiatry and Neurology
Certified, American Board of Adolescent Psychiatry
Clinical Professor of Psychiatry, Georgetown University Hospital

Appendix One

Recommended Resources

FINDING THE RIGHT DOCTOR

If you are trying to find a new doctor to better address your antidepressant side effects, I recommend a two-pronged approach.

Psychopharmacologist. You should see a psychopharmacologist, a physician (often a psychiatrist) who has expertise in prescribing mood-altering medications such as antidepressants. Psychopharmacologists can work with you by prescribing a new medication or changing the timing or dose of your medication.

The American Society of Clinical Psychopharmacology, Inc., is an association of physicians who specialize in the uses of these medications. Some of the members of this organization (myself included) have passed a rigorous exam on clinical psychopharmacology. The phone number is 212-268-4260. The address is P.O. Box 2257, New York, NY 10116.

The American Society of Clinical Psychopharmacology, Inc., can provide a list of psychopharmacologists in your area. Send a self-addressed, stamped (with ninety-nine cents postage) envelope to ASCP, P.O. Box 2257, New York, NY 10116. In addition to the referral list, you can request information about depression and a copy of the National Foundation for Depressive Illness (NAFDI) newsletter. The foundation requests a five-dollar donation to cover printing costs.

Functional medicine physician. Once you and your physician have determined that you are on the appropriate medication regimen, you need to find a physician who can determine if you have other medical problems (such as a food sensitivity or underactive thyroid) that may be causing side effects or lingering depression. If your physician is unwilling or unable to order the appropriate medical tests as outlined in Chapters 8 through 10 of this book, you should consider seeing a physician who practices functional medicine. Functional medicine includes physicians in various specialties that focus on restoring individual biochemical and metabolic balance. Practitioners of functional medicine employ laboratory tests to assess the various systems of the body: gastrointestinal, immune, endocrine (hormones), metabolic. They consider the body as an integrated whole rather than sets of isolated parts.

For more information on functional medicine, contact Health-Comm International, a private corporation dedicated to the development of functional medicine and nutrition. Call (800) 843-9660, or visit their Website at http://www.healthcomm.com.

Great Smokies Diagnostic Laboratory can also provide a list of functional medicine physicians in your area who use their laboratory services. Call (800) 522-4762 for a referral.

LABORATORIES

In Chapters 8 through 10 I recommend medical tests that may be appropriate for you depending on your symptoms and medical history. Since I have found that results of these tests may vary from lab to lab, here is a list of the facilities I use because they have provided reliable results. Moreover, some of the tests I recommend are performed only at specific labs. I realize that many managed care providers specify the labs that they will cover. Be aware that you may need to pay for some of these tests out of pocket.

Complete Blood Cell Count

American Medical Laboratory, Inc.
14225 Newbrook Drive
P.O. Box 10841
Chantilly, VA 20153-0841
(703) 802-6900

Thyroid Hormones
TSH, free T_4, free T_3

American Medical Laboratory, Inc.

Sex Hormones
(free testosterone, serum prolactin, luteinizing hormone, follicle-stimulating hormone, PSA)

American Medical Laboratory, Inc.

Adrenal Stress Index (ASI)

Diagnosis-Techs, Inc.
6620 South 192nd Place, No. J104
Kent, WA 98032
(800) 878-3787

Mineral Analysis of Red Blood Cells, Plasma, and Urine

Bay Area Laboratory Co-operative
(BALCO)
1520 Gilberth Road
Burlingame, CA 94010
(800) 777-7122

Comprehensive Digestive Stool Analysis (CDSA)

Great Smokies Diagnostic
Laboratory
Asheville, NC 28801-1074
(800) 522-4762

Liver Detoxification Profile

Great Smokies Diagnostic
Laboratory

Essential Fatty Acid Analysis

Great Smokies Diagnostic
Laboratory

Food Sensitivity Testing

Immuno Laboratories
1620 West Oakland Park Blvd.
Suite 300
Fort Lauderdale, FL 33311
(800) 231-9197

BOOKS AND VIDEOS

NUTRITION

FOOD AND MOOD BY ELIZABETH SOMER, M.A., R.D. (HENRY HOLT, 1995)

This book describes how certain nutrients in food improve energy levels, sleep patterns, memory, and attitude. Also discusses how all these improvements can help with weight management.

G-INDEX DIET BY RICHARD PODELL, M.D. (WARNER, 1993)

This book outlines an eating plan based on stabilizing blood-sugar levels by choosing carbohydrates that have a low glycemic index while mixing in an appropriate amount of protein. Has a large recipe section.

PROTEIN POWER BY MICHAEL R. EADES AND MARY DAN EADES (BANTAM, 1996)

This book describes "not a high protein" but "an adequate protein diet" that provides the appropriate ratio of protein to carbohydrates. Contains recipes fairly in line with the nutrition plan described in this book, although you need to steer away from any recipes containing chocolate, refined sugar, alcohol, or excess protein.

THE COMPLETE BOOK OF FITNESS BY THE EDITORS OF FITNESS MAGAZINE WITH KAREN ANDES (THREE RIVERS PRESS, 1999)

This book is an A-to-Z guide to all aspects of exercise—cardiovascular, stretches, and strength training. Contains a section on nutrition and preventing and recovering from injuries.

THE JOY OF FITNESS BY ED GAUT, CPFT (PIERPOINT-MARTIN, 1998)

The focus of this book is on making exercise fun. Contains a large section on play and incorporating play into your everyday life.

WEIGHT TRAINING FOR DUMMIES BY LIZ NEPORENT AND SUZANNE SCHLOSBERG (IDG BOOKS, 1997)

This book has plenty of easy-to-understand instruction for complete beginners, as well as information for those who have been training awhile. Helps design a program that's right for you by laying out basic principles of weight training and providing information on what you need to get started at home or at the gym. Includes photos and illustrations of exercises.

THE FIRM WORKOUT TAPES

This is a series of workout tapes that you can buy individually. Combines multiple dumbbell routines with aerobic floor work to give an aerobic workout while strength training. Some tapes incorporate step workouts into the routine.

KEYS TO WEIGHT TRAINING

This instructional video emphasizes free weights (not gym-type machines). Working from the larger muscle groups to the smaller, you'll create a progression of three complete routines.

REEBOK: AEROSTEP WITH GIN MILLER

This video provides a blend of step training and aerobic dance that continually shifts between step and floor aerobics.

TAE BO WITH BILLY BLANK

This video package presents a unique blend of tae kwon do, boxing, and aerobics set to a hip-hop beat. Comes as a four-tape set, which includes an instructional video and an eleven-minute short video for your busy days.

To obtain a free catalog of fitness videos, "The Complete Guide to Exercise Videos," contact Collage Exercise Video Specialists at (800) 433-6769.

PLEASURE, JOY, AND PLAY

LIGHTPOSTS FOR LIVING: THE ART OF CHOOSING A JOYFUL LIFE BY THOMAS KINKADE (WARNER, 1999)

This is an unusual book written by a renowned artist. It is a wonderful tool to use to achieve your goal of enhancing daily pleasures.

RELAXATION

BEYOND THE RELAXATION RESPONSE BY HERBERT BENSON, M.D., AND WILLIAM PROCTOR (TIMES, 1984)

THE COMPLETE BOOK OF RELAXATION TECHNIQUES BY JENNY SUTCLIFFE (PEOPLE'S MEDICAL SOCIETY, 1994)

THE MEDITATIVE MIND: THE VARIETIES OF MEDITATIVE EXPERIENCE BY DANIEL GOLEMAN (PUTNAM, 1996)

THE RELAXATION RESPONSE BY HERBERT BENSON, M.D., AND MIRIAM Z. KLIPPER (AVON, 1976)

This book describes how to achieve the relaxation response through breathing, muscle relaxation, and meditative focus. Incorporates Eastern techniques with Western medicine.

TRANSCENDENTAL MEDITATION

CREATING HEALTH: HOW TO WAKE UP THE BODY'S INTELLIGENCE BY DEEPAK CHOPRA (HOUGHTON MIFFLIN, 1995)

TM: TRANSCENDENTAL MEDITATION: A NEW INTRODUCTION TO MAHARISHI'S EASY, EFFECTIVE AND SCIENTIFICALLY PROVEN TECHNIQUE FOR PROMOTING BETTER HEALTH BY ROBERT ROTH (DONALD I. FINE, 1994)

THE TRANSCENDENTAL MEDITATION TM BOOK: HOW TO ENJOY THE REST OF YOUR LIFE BY DENISE DENNISTON (FAIRFIELD PRESS, 1986)

Appendix Two

Glycemic Index of Foods

All carbohydrates are not created equal. Although all are broken down by the body into glucose (the primary building block of carbohydrates), some are broken down much faster than others. These are known as high glycemic index foods (quick energy sources) because they cause an almost instantaneous rise in blood sugar. Unfortunately, the energy rush doesn't last long; blood-sugar levels plummet, causing an energy lull and perhaps more intense cravings for sugar.

Through laboratory studies researchers have identified which high-carbohydrate foods have a high glycemic index (thus cause a rapid rise in blood sugar), which have a low glycemic index (thus cause a slower rise in blood sugar), and which fall somewhere in between. These findings are summarized in the following lists of foods categorized by their glycemic indexes.

Source: K. Foster-Powell, *American Journal of Clinical Nutrition* 62, no. 4, October 1995: 871S–890S.

FOODS WITH A LOW GLYCEMIC INDEX
(BELOW 50 PERCENT)

These are the best carbohydrates.

Breads

Burgen soy lin
Burgen oat bran
Burgen honey loaf
Burgen mixed grain

Breakfast Cereals

Rice bran

Cereal Grains

Barley, pearled
Rye

Dairy Foods

Yogurt, artificially sweetened
and fruit sugar sweetened
Milk, regular, low-fat, skim

Fruit and Fruit Products

Cherries
Grapefruit
Apricots, dried

Legumes

Soybeans
Lentils, dried
Kidney beans
Butter beans
Lima beans

Chickpeas
Split peas
Dried peas
Peanuts and assorted nuts

Pasta

Spaghetti, protein enriched
Fettuccine, egg enriched

Sugar Sweeteners

Fructose

FOODS WITH A MEDIUM GLYCEMIC INDEX (50 TO 74 PERCENT)

Eat in moderate amounts (1 to 2 servings a day).

Bakery Products

Sponge cake
Banana cake, made with sugar

Breads

Barley kernel bread
Rye kernel bread
Mixed-grain bread
Oat bran bread
Pumpernickel

Breakfast Cereals

Kellogg's All-Bran Fruit 'n
Oats
Kellogg's Guardian
All-Bran

Cereal Grains

Wheat kernels
Rice, instant, boiled 1 minute
Bulgur
Rice, parboiled
Barley, cracked

Dairy Foods

Yogurt, unspecified
Ice cream, low-fat

Fruit and Fruit Products

Pear
Apple
Plum
Apple juice
Peach
Orange
Grapes

Pineapple juice
Grapefruit juice
Orange juice

Legumes

Navy beans
Pinto beans
Chickpeas, canned
Black-eyed peas
Romano beans
Baked beans, canned
Kidney beans, canned
Lentils, green, canned

Pasta

Vermicelli
Linguine
Spaghetti, whole-meal or
white

Ravioli, durum, meat-filled
Spirali, durum
Capellini
Macaroni
Instant noodles
Tortellini, cheese

Soups

Tomato soup
Lentil soup, canned

Sugar Sweeteners

Lactose

Vegetables

Yams
Peas, green
Carrots

Foods with a Moderately High Glycemic Index (75 to 100 percent)

Eat only on limited occasions (a few times a week).

Bakery Products

Cake, pound
Pastry
Pizza, cheese
Muffins
Cake, flan
Cake, angel food
Croissant
Crumpet

Breads

Pita bread, white
Hamburger bun

Wheat bread, high-fiber
Wheat bread, whole-meal
flour
Barley-flour bread
Rye-flour bread

Breakfast Cereals

Special K
Oat bran
Muesli
Shredded wheat
Nutri-Grain
Bran Chex

Life
Instant oatmeal

Cereal Grains

Wheat, quick-cooking
Buckwheat
Sweet corn
Rice, brown, wild, white
Couscous
Barley, rolled
Taco shells
Cornmeal

Dairy Foods

Ice cream, regular

Fruit and Fruit Products

Kiwifruit
Banana
Fruit cocktail
Mango
Apricots, fresh or canned
Raisins
Pineapple

Pasta

Spaghetti, durum
Macaroni and cheese, boxed
Gnocchi

Snack Foods

Potato chips
Popcorn
Oatmeal cookies
Shortbread
Arrowroot
Breton wheat crackers
Stoned wheat crackers

Soups

Split pea soup
Black bean soup
Green pea soup, canned

Sugar Sweeteners

Honey
High-fructose corn syrup
Sucrose (table sugar)

Vegetables

Sweet potato
Sweet corn
Potato, white
Potato, new
Beets

FOODS WITH A HIGH GLYCEMIC INDEX (100 PERCENT OR ABOVE)

Avoid these foods altogether.

Bakery Products

Donut
Waffle

Breads

Melba toast

Whole-wheat snack bread
(such as Wonder)
Bagel, white
Kaiser roll
Bread stuffing
French baguette

Breakfast Cereals

Cream of Wheat
Cheerios
Puffed wheat
Breakfast bars
Total
Corn bran
Crispix
Corn and Rice Chex
Rice Krispies

Cereal Grains

Millet
Rice, instant, boiled 6 minutes
Tapioca, boiled with milk

Fruit and Fruit Products

Watermelon

Snack Foods

Corn chips
Pretzels
Jelly beans
Graham wafers
Vanilla wafers
Water crackers
Rice cakes
Puffed crispbread

Sugar Sweeteners

Glucose
Glucose tablets
Maltodextrin
Maltose

Vegetables

French fries
Potato, mashed
Potato, baked
Parsnips
Pumpkin
Rutabaga

Appendix Three

Medical References

COMPREHENSIVE DIGESTIVE STOOL ANALYSIS, THE GUT, AND PSYCHIATRY

Caspary, W. F. "Physiology and pathophysiology of intestinal absorption." *American Journal of Clinical Nutrition,* 1992, 55: 299S–308S.

Gottschall, E. *Breaking the Vicious Cycle: Intestinal Health Through Diet.* Baltimore, Ontario: Kirkton Press Ltd., 1994.

Hoverstad, T. "The normal microflora and short-chain fatty acids." In Grubb, R., Midtvedt, T., and Norin, E., *The Regulatory and Protective Role of the Normal Microflora: Proceedings of the Fifth Bengt. E. Gustafsson Symposium,* vol. 52. New York: Stockton Press, 1989, 89–108.

Howitz, J., Schwartz, M. "Vitiligo, achlorhydria, and pernicious anemia." *Lancet,* 1971: 1331–34.

Hulst, R. R., Meyenfeldt, M. F., Soeters, P. B. "Glutamine: an essential amino acid for the gut." *Nutrition,* 1996, 12(11–12): S78–S81.

Hunter, J. O. "Food allergy—or enterometabolic disorder?" *Lancet,* 1991, 338: 495–96.

Lizko, N. N. "Stress and intestinal microflora." *Die Nahrung,* 1987, 31(5–6): 443–47.

Maki, M., Collin, P. "Coeliac disease." *Lancet,* 1997, 349: 1755–59.

Odds, F. C. *Candida and Candidosis: A Review and Bibliography,* 2nd ed. London: Bailliere Tindall, 1988, 71–83.

Olden, Kevin W. "A New Alliance Between Psychiatry and Gastroenterology." *Psychiatric Annals* 22(12): 596–97.

Rappaport, E. M. "Achlorhydria: associated symptoms and response to hydrochloric acid." *New England Journal of Medicine,* 1955, 25: 802–805.

Roberfroid, M. B. "Health benefits of non-digestible oligosaccharides." *Advances in Experimental and Medical Biology,* 1997, 427: 211–19.

Welbourne, T. C. "Increased plasma bicarbonate and growth hormone after oral glutamic acid." *American Journal of Nutrition,* 1995, 61(5): 1058–61.

DETOXIFICATION PROFILE

Bland, J. S., Bralley, J. A., Rigden, S. *Management of Chronic Fatigue Symptoms by Tailored Nutritional Intervention Using a Program Designed to Support Hepatic Detoxification.* Gig Harbor, WA: HealthComm, Inc., 1997.

Buist, R. A. "Chronic Fatigue Syndrome and Chemical Overload." 1988, 8(4): 173–75.

Costarella, L., Liska, D. J., Furlong, J., Lukaczer, D., Jones, D., Rountree, R., Larson Irwin, D. *Detoxification: A Clinical Monograph.* Institute for Functional Medicine, Inc., 1999.

Jost, G., Wahllander, A., von Mandach, U., Preisig, R. "Overnight salivary caffeine clearance: a liver function test suitable for routine use." *Hepatology,* 1987, 7(2): 338–44.

Krijgsheld, K. R., Mulder, G. L. "The availability of inorganic sulfate as a rate-limiting factor in the sulfation of zenobiotics in mammals *in vivo.*" In Mulder, G. L., et al., eds., *Sulfate Metabolism and Sulfate Conjugation.* London: Taylor and Francis, 1982, 59.

Levy, G. "Sulfate conjugation in drug metabolism: role of inorganic sulfate." *Federation Proc,* 1986, 45: 2235–40.

Liska, D., Lukaczer, D., Furlong, J. *Detoxification: A Clinical Monograph.* Jointly sponsored by the Postgraduate Institute for Medicine and the Institute for Functional Medicine, Inc., 1999.

Mulder, G. L., ed. *Conjugation Reactions in Drug Metabolism: An Integrated Approach.* London: Taylor and Francis, 1990.

Renner, E., Wietholtz, H., Huguenin, P., Arnaud, M. J., Preisig, R. "Caffeine: a model compound for measuring liver function." *Hepatology,* 1984, 4(1): 38–46.

Steventon, G. B., Heafield, M. T., Waring, R. H., Williams, A. C. "Xenobiotic metabolism in Parkinson's disease." *Neurology,* 1989, 39: 883–87.

Tong, S., Baghurst, P. A., Sawyer, M. G., Burns, J., McMichael, A. J. "Declining blood lead levels and changes in cognitive function during childhood: The Port Pirie Cohort study." *Journal of the American Medical Association,* 1998, 280(22): 1915–19.

ESSENTIAL FATTY ACIDS

Edwards, R., Peet, M., Shay, J., Horrobin, D. "Omega-3 polyunsaturated fatty acid levels in the diet and in red blood cell membranes of depressed patients." *Journal of Affective Disorders,* 1998, 48: 149–55.

Erasmus, U. *Fats and Oils: The Complete Guide to Fats and Oils in Health and Nutrition.* Vancouver, Canada: Alive Books, 1986.

Severus, W. E. "Omega-3 Fatty Acids—The Missing Link?" (letter to the editor). *Archives of General Psychiatry,* 1999, 56: 380.

Stoll, A. L., Severus, W. E., Freeman, M. P., et al. "Omega-3 fatty acids in bipolar disorder." *Archives of General Psychiatry,* 1999, 56: 407–12.

GLUCOSE HOMEOSTASIS

Berlin, I., Grimaldi, A., Landault, C., Cesselin, F., Puech, A. J. "Suspected post-prandial hypoglycemia is associated with beta-adrenergic hypersensitivity and emotional distress." *Journal of Clinical Endocrinology and Metabolism,* 1994, 79: 1428–33.

Cam, M. C., Li, W. M., McNeill, J. H. "Partial preservation of pancreatic beta-cells by vanadium: evidence for long-term amelioration of diabetes." *Metabolism,* 1997, 46: 769–78.

Sprietsma, J. E., Schuitemaker, G. E. "Diabetes can be prevented by reducing insulin production." *Medical Hypotheses,* 1994, 42: 15–23.

Spring, B., Chiodo, J., Harden, M., Bourgeois, M., Mason, J., Lutherer, L. "Psychobiological effects of carbohydrates." *Journal of Clinical Psychiatry,* 1989, 50(5): S27–S33.

Winokur, A., Maislin, G., Phillips, J. L., Amsterdam, J. D. "Insulin resistance after oral glucose tolerance testing in patients with major depression." *American Journal of Psychiatry,* 1988, 145(3): 325–30.

HERBAL AND NATURAL REMEDIES FOR DEPRESSION

Bell, K. M., Plon, L., Bunney, W. E., Jr., Potkin, S. G. "S-adenosylmethionine treatment of depression: a controlled clinical trial." *American Journal of Psychiatry,* 1988, 145(9): 1110–14.

Kagan, B. L., et al. "Oral S-adenosylmethionine in depression: a randomized, double-blind, placebo-controlled trial." *American Journal of Psychiatry,* 1990, 147(5): 591–95.

Kleijnen, J., Knipschild, P. "Ginkgo biloba." *Lancet,* 1992, 340: 1136–39.

Krieglstein, J., Ausmeir, F. "Neuroprotective effects of ginkgo biloba constituents." *European Journal of Pharmacological Science,* 1995, 3: 39–48.

Linde, K., Ramirez, G., Murlow, C. D., Pauls, A., Weidenhammer, W., Melchart, D. "St John's wort for depression: an overview and meta-analysis of randomised clinical trials." *British Medical Journal,* 1996, 313: 253–58.

Rosenbaum, J. L., et al. "The antidepressant potential of oral S-adenosyl-l-methionine." *Acta Psychiatry Scandinavia,* May 1990, 81(5): 432–36.

Volz, H-P. "Controlled clinical trials of hypericum extracts in depressed patients: an overview." *Pharmacopsychiatry,* 1997, 30: 72–76.

IMMUNITY

Brostoff, J., Scadding, G. K. "Immunological and clinical aspects of food allergy." *Italian Journal of Medicine,* 1985, 1: 2-3.

Calabrese, J. R., Kling, M. A., Gold, P. W. "Alterations in immunocompetence during stress, bereavement, and depression: focus on neuroendocrine regulation." *American Journal of Psychiatry,* 1987, 144(9): 1123–34.

Chandra, R. K. "Graying of the immune system: can nutrient supplements improve immunity in the elderly?" (commentary). *Journal of the American Medical Association,* 1997, 277(17): 1398–99.

Connor, T. J., Leonard, B. E. "Minireview: depression, stress, and immunological activation: the role of cytokines in depressive disorders." *Life Sciences,* 1998, 62(7): 583–606.

DeSimoni, M. G., Imeri, L. "Cytokine-neurotransmitter interactions in the brain." *Biological Signals and Receptors,* 1998, 7: 33–44.

Evans, D. L. "Circulating natural killer cell phenotypes in men and women with major depression: relation to cytotoxic activity and severity of depression." *Archives of General Psychiatry,* 1992, 49(5): 388–95.

Glaser, R., Rabin, B., Chesney, M., Cohen, S., Natelson, B. "Stress-induced immunomodulation: implications for infectious diseases?" *Journal of the American Medical Association,* 1999, 281(24): 2268–70.

Goujon, E., Laye, S., Dantzer, P., Dantzer, R. "Regulation of cytokine gene expression in the central nervous system by glucocorticoids: mechanisms and functional consequences." *Psychoneuroendocrinology,* 1997, 22 (supplement 1): S75–S80.

Maes, M. "Lower serum dipeptidyl peptidase IV activity in treatment resistant major depression: relationships with immune-inflammatory markers." *Psychoneuroendocrinology,* 1997, 22(2): 65–78.

Maes, M., Bosmans, E., Meltzer, H., Scharpe, S., Suy, E. "Interleukin-1 beta: a putative mediator of HPA axis activity in major depression?" *American Journal of Psychiatry,* 1993, 150(8): 1189–93.

Marx, C. "Regulation of adrenocortical function by cytokines—relevance for immune endocrine interaction." *Hormone and Metabolism Research,* 1998, 30(6–7): 416–20.

Muller, N., Ackenheil, M. "Psychoneuroimmunology and cytokine action in the CNS: implications for psychiatric disorders." *Progress in Neuro-Psychopharmacology and Biological Psychiatry,* 1998, 22: 1–33.

Neiman, D. C. "Exercise immunology: practical applications." *International Journal of Sports Medicine,* 1997, 18 (supplement 1): S91–S100.

Restak, R. M. "The brain, depression, and the immune system." *Journal of Clinical Psychiatry,* 1989, 50(5): S23–S25.

Sampson, H. A. "Food allergy." *Journal of the American Medical Association,* 278 (22): 1888–94.

Sigal, L. H., Yacov, R. *Immunology and Inflammation: Basic Mechanisms and Clinical Consequences.* New York: McGraw-Hill, 1994, chapters 23 and 24.

Song, C., Dinan, T., Leonard, B. E. "Changes in immunoglobulin, complement and acute phase protein levels in the depressed patients and normal controls." *Journal of Affective Disorders,* 1994, 30: 283–88.

Stein, M. "Stress, depression, and the immune system." *Journal of Clinical Psychiatry,* 1989, 50(5): S35–S40.

Weiss, J. M., Sundar, S. K., Becker, K. J., Cierpiel, M. A. "Behavioral and neural influences on cellular immune responses: effects of stress and interleukin-1." *Journal of Clinical Psychiatry,* 1989, 50(5): S43–S53.

Woiciechowsky, C., Schoning, B., Daberkow, N., Asche, K., Stoltenburg, G., Lanksch, W. R., Volk, H. D. "Brain-IL-1 beta induces local inflammation but systemic anti-inflammatory response through stimulation of both hypothalamic-pituitary-adrenal axis and sympathetic nervous system." *Brain Research,* 1999, 816(2): 563–71.

METALS, MINERALS, AND ASSESSMENT OF LEVELS

Bulai, Z. J. "Clinical and biochemical abnormalities in people heterozygous for hemochromatosis." *New England Journal of Medicine,* 1996, 335: 1799–1805.

Cutler, P. "Iron overload and psychiatric illness." *Canadian Journal of Psychiatry,* 1994, 39: 8–11.

Feifel, D. "Iron overload among a psychiatric outpatient population." *Journal of Clinical Psychiatry,* 1997, 58: 74–78.

Foo, S. C., Khoo, N. Y., Heng, A., Chua, L. H., Chia, S. E., Ong, C. N., Ngim, C. H., Jeyaratnam, J. "Metals in hair as biological indices for exposure." *International Archives of Occupational and Environmental Health,* 1993, 65: S83–S86.

Jenkins, D. W., Santolucito, J. A. "Biological monitoring of toxic trace metals, volume 1: Biological monitoring and surveillance." Report from the Office of Research and Development, U.S. Environmental Protection Agency, September 1980.

Kimura, K. "Role of essential trace elements in the disturbance of carbohydrate metabolism." *Nippon Rinsho,* 1996, 54 (supplement 1): 79–84.

Laker, M. "On determining trace element levels in man: the uses of blood and hair." *Lancet,* 1982: 260–61.

Maes, M., Vandoolaeghe, E., Demedts, P., Wauters, A., Meltzer, H. Y., Altamura, C., Desnyder, R. "Lower serum zinc in major depression is a sensitive marker of treatment resistance and of the immune/inflammatory response in that illness." *Biological Psychiatry,* 1997, 42 (supplement 5): 349–58.

Maugh, T. H. "Hair: a diagnostic tool to complement blood serum and urine." *Science,* 1978, 202: 1271–73.

McLeod, M. N., Gaynes, B. N., Golden, R. N. "Chromium potentiation of antidepressant pharmacotherapy for dysthymic disorder in 5 patients." *Journal of Clinical Psychiatry,* 1999, 60: 237–40.

Narang, R., Gupta, K., Narang, A., Singh, R. "Levels of copper and zinc in depression." *Indian Journal of Physiological Pharmacology,* 35 (supplement 4): 272–74.

Naylor, G. J. "Vanadium and manic depressive psychosis." *Nutrition and Health,* 1984, 3: 79–85.

Pfeiffer, C., Braverman, E. "Zinc, the brain, and behavior." *Biological Psychiatry,* 1982, 17 (supplement 4): 513–32.

Pfeiffer, C. C. "Elementary, dear Watson!" *Biology Psychiatry,* 1987, 22: 805–806.

Smith, B. L. "Cardiovascular risk as related to an element pattern in hair." *Trace Elements in Medicine,* 1987, 4(3): 131–33.

Yung, C. Y. "A Synopsis on Metals in Medicine and Psychiatry." *Pharmacology, Biochemistry and Behavior,* 1984, 21 (supplement 1): 41–47.

MISCELLANEOUS

Goodman, A. "Organic unity theory: the mind-body problem revisited." *American Journal of Psychiatry,* 148(5): 553–63.

Kupfer, D. J., Frank, E., Perel, J. M., Cornes, C., Mallinger, A. G., Thase, M. E., McEachran, A. B., Grochocinski, V. J. "Five-year outcome for maintenance therapies in recurrent depression." *Archives of General Psychiatry,* 1992, 49: 769–73.

Martin, M. J. "A brief review of organic diseases masquerading as functional illness." *Hospital and Community Psychiatry,* 1983, 34(4): 328–32.

Neumeister, A., Turner, E. H., Matthews, J. R., et al. "Effects of tryptophan depletion vs. catecholamine depletion in patients with seasonal affective disorder in remission with light therapy." *Archives of General Psychiatry,* 1998, 55: 524–30.

ORGANIC FOODS AND PESTICIDES

Guillette, E. A., Meza, M. M. "An anthropological approach to the evaluation of preschool children exposed to pesticides in Mexico." *Environmental Health Perspectives,* 1998, 106(6): 347–53.

Raloff, J. "Beyond estrogens: why unmasking hormone-mimicking pollutants proves so challenging." *Science News,* 1995, 148: 44–46.

Raloff, J. "Picturing pesticides' impacts on kids." *Science News,* 1998, 153.

Smith, B. L. "Organic foods vs. supermarket foods: element levels." *Journal of Applied Nutrition,* 1993, 45(1): 35–39.

Worthington, V. "Effects of agricultural methods on nutritional quality: a comparison of organic with conventional crops." *Alternative Therapies,* 1998, 4: 58–69.

REWARD AND PLEASURE

Robbins, T. W., and Everitt, B. J. "Neurobehavioral mechanisms of reward and motivation." *Current Opinion in Neurology,* 1996, 6: 228–36.

SALIVARY CORTISOL, DHEA, AND ADRENAL FUNCTION

Granger, D. A., Schwartz, E. B., Booth, A., Curran, M., Zakaria, D. "Assessing dehydroepiandrosterone in saliva: a simple radioimmunoassay for use in studies of children, adolescents, and adults." *Psychoneuroendocrinology,* 1999, 24: 567–79.

Guechot, J., Lepine, J. P., Cohen, C., Fiet, J., Lemperiere, T., Dreux, C. "Simple laboratory test of neuroendocrine disturbance in depression: 11 p.m. saliva cortisol." *Biological Psychiatry, Neuropsychobiology,* 1987, 18: 1–4.

Kahn, J-P., Rubinow, D. R., Davis, C. L., Kling, M., Post, R. M. "Salivary cortisol: a practical method for evaluation of adrenal function." *Biological Psychiatry,* 1988, 23: 335–49.

Laudat, M. H., Cerdas, S., Fournier, C., Guiban, D., Guilhaume, B., Lupton, J. P. "Salivary cortisol measurement: a practical approach to assess pituitary-adrenal function." *Journal of Clinical Endocrinology and Metabolism,* 1988, 66: 343.

Marx, C. "Regulation of adrenocortical function by cytokines—relevance for immune endocrine interaction." *Hormone and Metabolism Research,* 1998, 30(6–7): 416–20.

Nemeroff, C. B. "Clinical significance of psychoendocrinology in psychiatry: focus on thyroid and adrenal." *Journal of Clinical Psychiatry,* 1989, 50(5): S13–S20.

Ozasa, H., Kita, M., Inoue, T., Mori, T. "Plasma dehydroepiandrosterone-to-cortisol ratios as an indicator of stress in gynecologic patients." *Gynecologic Oncology,* 1990, 37: 178–82.

Raber, J. "Detrimental effects of chronic hypothalamic-pituitary-adrenal axis activation. From obesity to memory deficits." *Molecular Neurobiology,* 1998, 18(1): 1–22.

Riad-Fahmy, D. "Steroids in saliva for assessing endocrine function." *Endocrine Society,* 3: 367–95.

Rubin, R. T., Phillips, J. J., Sadow, T. F., McCracken, J. T. "Adrenal gland volume in major depression: increase during the depressive episode and decrease with successful treatment." *Archives of General Psychiatry,* 1995, 52: 213–18.

Swinkels, M.J.W., Ross, H. A., Smals, A.G.H., Benraad, Th. J. "Concentrations of total and free dehydroepiandrosterone in plasma and dehydroepiandrosterone in saliva of normal and hirsute women under basal conditions and during administration of dexamethasone/synthetic corticotropin." *Clinical Chemistry,* 1990, 36(12): 2042–46.

Tunn, S., Mollmann, H., Barth, J., Derendorf, H., Krieg, M. "Simultaneous measurement of cortisol in serum and saliva after different forms of cortisol administration." *Clinical Chemistry*, 1992, 38(8): 1491–94.

Vining, R. F. "Salivary cortisol: a better measure of adrenal cortical function than serum cortisol." *Annals of Clinical Biochemistry*, 20: 329–35.

Walker, R. F. "Salivary cortisol determinations in the assessment of adrenal activity." *Frontiers in Oral Physiology*, 1984, 5: 33–50.

SEXUAL DYSFUNCTION AND REPRODUCTIVE HORMONES

Becker, A. J., Christian, G. S., Machtens, S., Schultheiss, D., Hartmann, U., Truss, M., Jonas, U. "Oral phentolamine as treatment for erectile dysfunction." *Journal of Urology*, 1998, 159: 1214–16.

Bergeron, R., de Montigny, C., Debonnel, G. "Potentiation of neuronal NMDA response induced by dehydroepiandrosterone and its suppression by progesterone: effects mediated via sigma receptors." *Journal of Neuroscience*, 1996, 16: 1193–202.

Ernst, E., Pittler, M. H. "Yohimbine for erectile dysfunction: a systematic review and meta-analysis of randomized clinical trials." *Journal of Urology*, 1998, 159(2): 433–36.

Fava, M., Rankin, M., Alpert, J., Nierenberg, A., Worthington, J. "An open trial of sildenafil in antidepressant-induced sexual dysfunction." *Psychotherapy and Psychosomatics*, 1998, 67: 328–31.

Fisher, S. "Postmarketing surveillance by patient self-monitoring: preliminary data for sertraline versus fluoxetine." *Journal of Clinical Psychiatry*, 1995, 56: 288–96.

Gelenberg, A. J. "Sex steroids and psychiatric symptoms." *Biological Therapies in Psychiatry Newsletter*, 1998, 21(12): 49–50.

Goldstein, I., Lue, T. F., Padma-Nathan, H. "Oral sildenafil in the treatment of erectile dysfunction." *New England Journal of Medicine*, 1998, 338: 1397–404.

Gunby, P. "Prostate detection possibility." *Journal of the American Medical Association*, 1999, 281(24): 2274.

Nurnberg, G. H., Lauriello, J., Hensley, P. L., Parker, L. M., Keith, S. "Sildenafil for iatrogenic serotonergic antidepressant medication–induced sexual dysfunction in 4 patients." *Journal of Clinical Psychiatry*, 1999, 60(1): 33–35.

Park, K., Moreland, Goldstein, I., Atala, A., Traish, A. "Sildenafil inhibits phosphodiesterase type 5 in human clitoral corpus cavernosum smooth muscle." *Biochemical and Biophysical Research Communications*, 1998, 249: 612–17.

Segraves, R. T. "Antidepressant-induced sexual dysfunction." *Journal of Clinical Psychiatry,* 1998, 59: S48–S54.

"Side effects: use creative solutions to battle sexual side effects of SSRI's." *Psychopharmacology Update,* 1998, 9(3).

Stahl, S. "How psychiatrists can build new therapies for impotence." *Journal of Clinical Psychiatry,* 1998, 59(2): 47–48.

Sternbach, H. "Age-associated testosterone decline in men: clinical issues for psychiatry." *American Journal of Psychiatry,* 1998, 155(10): 1310–17.

Sussman, N. "The role of antidepressants in sexual dysfunction." *Journal of Clinical Psychiatry,* monograph, 17, no. 1, March 1999: 9–14.

Thompson, D. "Patterns of antidepressant use and their relation to costs of care." *American Journal of Managed Care,* 1996, 2(9): 1239–46.

Winters, S. J. "Androgens: endocrine physiology and pharmacology." In *Anabolic Steroid Abuse,* G. C. Lin, L. Erinoff, eds. Research Monograph 102. Rockville, Md.: U.S. Department of Health and Human Services, Public Health Service, Alcohol, Drug Abuse, and Mental Health Administration, National Institute on Drug Abuse, 1990.

THYROID AXIS AND AFFECTIVE DISORDERS

Bunevicius, R. "Effects of thyroxine as compared with thyroxine plus triiodothyronine in patients with hypothyroidism." *New England Journal of Medicine,* 1999, 340(6): 424–29.

Bunevicius, R., Kazanavicius, G., Telksnys, A. "Thyrotropin response to TRH stimulation in depressed patients with autoimmune thyroiditis." *Biology in Psychiatry,* 1994, 36: 543–47.

Clary, C., Harrison, W. "Spokespersons for Pfizer Laboratories reply" (letter). *New England Journal of Medicine,* 1997, 337: 1011.

Cooper, D. S. "Thyroid hormone, osteoporosis, and estrogen." *Journal of the American Medical Association,* 1994, 271(16): 1283–84.

Haggerty, J. J., Evans, D. L., Golden, R. N., et al. "The presence of antithyroid antibodies in affective and non-affective psychiatric disorders." *Biology in Psychiatry,* 1990, 27: 51.

Haggerty, J. J., Garbutt, J. C., Evans, D. L., et al. "Subclinical hypothyroidism: a review of neuro-psychiatric aspects." *International Journal of Psychiatry Medicine,* 1990, 20(2): 193.

Hauser, P. "Attention deficit–hyperactivity disorder in people with generalized resistance to thyroid hormone." *New England Journal of Medicine,* 328(14): 997–1001.

Joffe, Russell T. "The use of thyroid supplements to augment antidepressant medication." *Journal of Clinical Psychiatry,* 1998, 59 : S26–S29.

Marangell, L. B., Ketter, T. A., George, M. S., Pazzaglia, P. J., Callahan, A. M., Parekh, P., Andreason, P. J., Horwitz, B., Herscovitch, P., Post, R. M. "Inverse relationship of peripheral thyrotropin-stimulating hormone levels to brain activity in mood disorders." *American Journal of Psychiatry,* 1997, 154: 224–30.

McCowen, K., Spark, R. "Elevated serum thyrotropin in thyroxine-treated patients with hypothyroidism given sertraline" (letter). *New England Journal of Medicine,* 1997, 337: 1010–11.

O'Hara, H. W., Schlechte, J. A., Lewis, D. A., et al. "Prospective study of postpartum blues: biological and psychosocial factors." *Archives of General Psychiatry,* 1991 48(9): 801.

Schneider, D. L., Barrett-Connor, E. L., Morton, D. J. "Thyroid hormone use and bone mineral density in elderly women." *Journal of the American Medical Association,* 1994, 271(16): 1245–48.

Toft, A. "Thyroid hormone replacement—one hormone or two?" (editorial). *New England Journal of Medicine,* 1999, 340: 469–70.

VITAMIN B$_{12}$, FOLATE, AND PSYCHIATRY

Chary, T. K., Laundy, M., Bottiglieri, T., Chanarin, I., Reynolds, E. H., Toone, B. "Red cell folate concentrations in psychiatric patients." *Journal of Affective Disorders,* 1990, 19(3): 207–13.

Fava, M. "Folate, vitamin B$_{12}$, and homocysteine in major depressive disorder." *American Journal of Psychiatry,* 1997, 154(3): 426–28.

Fine, E. J., Soria, E. D. "Myths about vitamin B$_{12}$ deficiency." *Southern Medical Journal,* 1991, 84(12): 1475–81.

Guttormsen, A. B., Schneede, J., Ueland, P. M., Refsum, H. "Kinetics of total plasma homocysteine in subjects with hyperhomocysteinemia due to folate or cobalamin deficiency." *American Journal of Clinical Nutrition,* 1996, 63: 194–202.

Lindenbaum, J., Healton, E. B., Savage, D. G., et al. "Neuropsychiatric disorders caused by cobalamin deficiency in the absence of anemia or macrocytosis." *New England Journal of Medicine,* 1988, 318: 1720–28.

Mischoulon, D. "The role of folate in major depression: mechanisms and clinical implications." *American Society of Clinical Psychopharmacology Progress Notes,* 1996, 7(2): 4–5.

Robinson, K., Mayer, E. L., Miller, D. P., Green, R., van Lente, F., Gupta, A., Kottke-Marchant, K., Savon, S. R., Selhub, J., Nissen, S. E., Kutner, M., Topol, E. J., Jacobsen, D. W. "Hyperhomocysteinemia and low pyridoxal phosphate, common and independent reversible risk factors for coronary artery disease." *Circulation,* 1995, 92: 2825–30.

Stabler, S. P., Lindenbaum, J., Allen, R. H. "The use of homocysteine and other metabolites in the specific diagnosis of vitamin B-12 deficiency, colloquium: homocyst(e)ine, vitamins and arterial occlusive diseases." *American Institute of Nutrition,* 1996, 1266S–1272S.

Sumner, A. E., Chin, M. M., Abraham, J. L., Berry, G. T., Gracely, E. J., Allen, R. H., Stabler, S. P. "Elevated methylamalonic acid and total homocysteine levels show high prevalence of vitamin B_{12} deficiency after gastric surgery." *Annals of Internal Medicine,* 1996, 124: 469–76.

Toh, B.-H., Van Driel, I. R., Gleeson, P. A. "Pernicious anemia." *New England Journal of Medicine,* 1997, 337: 1441–48.

Williams, R. H., Maggiore, J. A. "Hyperhomocysteinemia, pathogenesis, clinical significance, laboratory assessment, and treatment." *Laboratory Medicine,* 1999, 30(7): 468–75.

WEIGHT GAIN

Baldwin, D. S., Birtwistle, J. "The side effect burden associated with drug treatment of panic disorder." *Journal of Clinical Psychiatry,* 1998, 59 (8): S39–S44.

Medina, J. "The genes of human appetite." *Psychiatric Times,* May 1998, 37–39.

Stahl, S. M. "Neuropharmacology of obesity: my receptors made me eat it." *Journal of Clinical Psychiatry,* 1998, 59 (9): 447–48.

Sussman, N., Ginsberg, D. "Weight gain associated with SSRI's." *Primary Psychiatry,* January 1998, 28–39.

Acknowledgments

Writing a book is the closest I will ever come, I think, to giving birth. It's painful, always seems to require one more push, is, in the end, clearly satisfying, and for some reason, the pain is easily forgotten, but quickly remembered. Unlike giving birth, however, conceiving and writing a book of this nature requires more than two people.

As always, were it not for my family—my dedicated and supportive wife, Mindy, who has been with me from Brooklyn to Buffalo and whose support has been pivotal, my light-filled children, Adam, Joshua, and Caroline, my genetically well-endowed parents, Caroll and Joe, my sibling rivals, brothers Harold and Nathan, and my irrepressible, smiling sister, Marilyn—I would not have been neurotic enough to go into psychiatry in the first place, nor would I have been supported enough to achieve very much of anything. The support, skills, and dilemmas these people have given me have been the sine qua non of my career.

In the mid-1980s, I was very fortunate to get to know my friend and trainer, David Sanchez. From my early racquetball days, when he taught me the art of that sport, to the more recent years of supporting my own physical renewal, David has always been an encouraging teacher. I doubt that this book could have been written without his influence.

Sometimes it seems that life sends someone your way at just the right time. Such is the case with my very good friend, Erwin Adler, or, as I affectionately think of him, "the man with the bike." Erwin's influence is woven throughout much of this book, as he has taught me the art of balancing both bike and life.

As fate would have it, I ran into Jodi Jaffe at the health club one day in 1997, and we began schmoozing. I mentioned to Jodi—an author herself—that I had some ideas for a book (I had the urge to give birth again), and Jodi generously provided me with the name of her friend and excellent book designer, Mary Challinor, who screened my idea before sending me on to the big guy, Josh Horwitz of Living Planet Press.

Josh Horwitz is the living embodiment of professionalism, responsibility, and, in times of difficulty, tactfulness. It is clear to me that more than anyone, this book would not exist without Josh's partnership. I consider myself very fortunate to have worked with a true professional such as Josh.

After Josh and I worked out the details, we put together a proposal, and with the help of Gail Ross, our agent, we set up fifteen meetings in New York—all in two days—with publishing houses. Gail gently and playfully guided me through the July heat and the repetitive presentations of the book's theme to each publishing house, and gave me the inside scoop on the subtle differences among the different houses. All along she encouraged me. (I can still hear her calm and even voice: "Bob, you're doing great.")

When I met with my editor, Patty Gift, Tina Constable (then the very pregnant publicity director), and Steve Ross, the editorial director at Crown, there was a clear chemistry. Since then, Patty has been a wonderful editor and supportive cheerleader, unwavering in her excitement about this book, and the purveyor of wonderful ideas.

Given my numerous responsibilities to my family, my patients, my teaching at Georgetown University Hospital, and my lecturing to other mental health professionals, it was clear to Josh that unlike my first book, I would need a writer who could accurately capture my ideas and voice on paper. Debbie Kotz did this quite well.

During my training at the National Institute of Mental Health, I was most fortunate to get to know Norman Rosenthal. A supreme researcher and innovative thinker, Norm has made a tremendous contribution to the lives of countless people by the identification and study of seasonal affective disorder (SAD) and his subsequent discovery of the efficacy of light therapy in this condition. Our friendship has blossomed and deepened over the years, and his kind words in the foreword are echoed by my respect for him.

In my journey through psychiatry, one person has been there from the very first moment—my dear friend, psychiatric brother, and colleague Rick Fernandez. If there are such things as past lives, Rick and

I have had several together. More likely, I have decided, our neuroses interconnect exceptionally well, as do our senses of humor and dedication to and love of psychiatry. Rick was generous enough to take time out from his family, busy practice, teaching at the University of Medicine and Dentistry in New Jersey, and volunteering on the New Jersey State Board of Medicine to review this manuscript for inaccuracies. But, as the author, I must ruefully take responsibility for any mistakes that may have found their way into these pages.

Finally, many thanks to both Linda Epstein and Dina Najjar for their administrative support and help in making this book possible. The timing of their arrival in my life was impeccable.

These, then, are the essential people who have contributed to this book, and they have my very deepest appreciation.

Index